Risk Management in Medicine

Walter Merkle

Editor

Risk Management
in Medicine

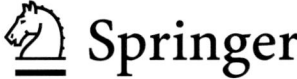 Springer

Editor
Walter Merkle, MD
Riskmanager in Medicine
Specialist in Urology
Management Expert for Hospitals (VWA)
German Diagnostic Clinic – Helios Clinic
Wiesbaden
Germany

ISBN 978-3-662-47406-8   ISBN 978-3-662-47407-5   (eBook)
DOI 10.1007/978-3-662-47407-5

Library of Congress Control Number: 2015958084

Springer Heidelberg New York Dordrecht London

Printed on acid-free paper

Springer-Verlag GmbH Berlin Heidelberg is part of Springer Science+Business Media (www.springer.com)

Preface

Risk Management in Hospitals – New subject or just new wine in old bottles?

Both are correct. Risk management as principle is a well-known tool, but currently not well used in hospitals.

Industrial enterprises have been developing risk management tools for decades. Motorola was the first company to start with systemic analysis as to why some procedures went wrong. It was shown that not Motorola was dealing with a problematic business, but is working with people – meaning with its staff.

Where people are working, mistakes and failures are common.

Errare humanum est – hundreds of years ago ancient Rome already knew this.

The systemic approach by Motorola and others showed that there is a baseline level of human-caused failures independent of the individual and independent of the business or procedure.

At the end of the last century, the Harvard Medical Study demonstrated that in medicine there is also a baseline level of 3 % failures in all medical procedures – what a surprise!? Really?

Meanwhile some efforts are taken analyzing the specific details in medicine with focus on hospitals.

This book will refer the current status of the details which now firm under the title of Risk Management.

Reducing risk in patient treatment is as ethically as economically justifiable.

The cause is simple – repair of wrong treatment costs additional money and the health of the patient as well. Furthermore, problems with the law might occur if something went wrong not only by accident but by malpractice of doctors and staff. This all together will cost a large amount of money and the reputation of the hospital.

Thus, total successful risk management does cost money to install, but it definitely saves more money than it costs, and patients are healthier.

There is no better win-win situation for everybody.

How does this work?

This textbook will demonstrate in every chapter why we make some mistakes, although we do not want to do so, and how to protect everybody – patients, doctors, and hospital administration (and insurance companies) against human failures.

The German issue was published successfully in February 2014.

As editor of this textbook, I am very pleased that my authors are more than willing to write the international issue which you hold in your hands.

Main parts of the German version are also part of the international textbook, but of course important chapters are written newly under the broader sight of Europe and the USA. Especially the law chapters had to be adjusted because of country-specific medical laws.

I therefore thank my old friend Prof. Joseph Smith Jr., Chairman of Urology at Vanderbilt University, for supporting the international version and assisting in writing parts under the specific US sight. Additionally I thank Dr. Rybak spontaneously for accepting my invitation in contributing with the European law chapter.

And last but not least I am grateful to my publisher Springer in Heidelberg, New York, and London for accepting my idea to publish an international version of our risk management textbook. The professional work of this publisher is invaluable and guarantees good quality.

Wiesbaden, Germany   Walter Merkle

Contents

Contributors

Editor

Walter Merkle, MD Riskmanager in Medicine Specialist in Urology, Management Expert for Hospitals (VWA), German Diagnostic Clinic – Helios Clinic, Wiesbaden, Germany

Contributors

Cord-H. Becker ATS Aviation Training Support, Wiesbaden, Germany

Sigrid Blehle, MD, MBA Köhn und Kollegen, Munich, Germany

Eugen H. Bühle Bühle hpm-Consult GmbH, Human Performance Management, Herrsching, Germany

Roger Roman Dmochowski, MD, MMHC, FACS Department of Urologic Surgery, Vanderbilt University, Nashville, TN, USA

A. Erdmann Wirtschaftsjurist (Univ. Bayreuth), Munich, Germany

Achim Göbel AirColleg GmbH, Weilmünster, Germany

Andreas Goepfert, MD Vorstand, ANregiomed, Ansbach, Germany

Dieter Hensel ATS Aviation Training Servies, Kriftel, Germany

Patrik Herrscher Leiter Dienstleistungszentrum Qualitäts- und Risikomanagement, ANregiomed, Ansbach, Germany

Roland H. Kaiser, MD Ärztlicher Direktor, Landesärztekammer Hessen, Frankfurt, Germany

Michael Keese, MD Klinik für Gefäßchirurgie und Endovascularchirurgie, Klinikum der Goethe-Universität, Frankfurt, Germany

Stephan Krempel Fachanwalt für Medizinrecht, Saarbrücken, Germany

Rainer Riedel, MD Institut für Medizin-Ökonomie, Medizinische Versorgungsforschung – iMÖV, Köln, Germany

Dirk-Matthias Rose, MD, PhD Institut für Lehrergesundheit am Institut für, Arbeits-, Sozial- und Umweltmedizin, Universitätsmedizin der Johannes-Gutenberg-Universität Mainz, Mainz, Germany

Christian Rybak, LLD Wirtschaftsjurist (Univ. Bayreuth), Munich, Germany

Aliki Schmieder, MA Masterstudiengang Medizinökonomie, RFH Köln, Köln, Germany

Thomas Schmitz-Rixen, MD, PhD Klinik für Gefäß- und Endovascularchirurgie und des universitären, Wundzentrums der Goethe-Universität, Chefarzt der Gefäßchirurgie am Hospital zum, Heiligen Geist gGmbH Frankfurt, Frankfurt, Germany

Sonja Sieger TÜV PROFiCERT-Lead Auditorin, TÜV Technische Überwachung Hessen GmbH, Managementsysteme, Darmstadt, Germany

Joseph A. Smith, MD Department of Urologic Surgery, Vanderbilt University, Nashville, TN, USA

C.J. Stimson, MD, JD Department of Urologic Surgery, Vanderbilt University Medical Center, Nashville, TN, USA

Regine Töpfer, MA Executive Coach, Rehnocken 67, Witten, Germany

Nina Walter, MA St. Leiterin Stabsstelle Qualitätssicherung, Versorgungsmanagement und Gesundheitsökonomie, Landesärztekammer Hessen, Frankfurt, Germany

R.A. Patrick Weidinger Abteilungsleiter, Deutsche Ärzteversicherung Aktiengesellschaft, Wiesbaden, Germany

Why We Do Wrong Although We Want to Do Right

Walter Merkle

Abstract

The question why we make mistakes although we want to do right is the main source to start risk management.

Mistakes and faults are mostly caused by principles owned by everybody. Thus it is important to find out how people act when making things wrongly. The overwhelming amount of these mistakes can happen to everybody and are not caused individually.

The principles of these processes and how to learn from these insights are discussed in this chapter. Technical aspects (e.g., zero-failure technique), psychological aspects (e.g., mobbing), solution techniques (e.g., peer reviews), and further solutions are put into a structured context.

1.1 Introduction

First of all, there is nobody who's happy to make mistakes.

And therefore nobody wants to admit to having made a mistake.

Thus, failures are covered by silence.

Consequently systemic failure will not be detected, and every single person will make the same mistake again; there's no learning process.

Everybody knows that there are systemic and principle failures independently from the person to make the mistake. Logically it seems to be possible to prevent those failures by training and information about pitfalls, etc.

However – an individual bottom level of failures will remain because we all are human beings. And also these individual failures can be reduced to an absolute minimum by intelligent support systems.

Altogether there is only one absolutely mandatory principle to accept – we all, youngsters as well as highly trained and experienced experts, will make mistakes our whole life. We all sit in the same boat.

Thus we all have to learn the tools to reduce the imminent risks. We all can learn from each other – but we have to do it!

The ethos of doctors and all medical staff fits together with the patient's claim to work correctly.

W. Merkle, MD
Riskmanager in Medicine Specialist in Urology,
Management Expert for Hospitals (VWA),
German Diagnostic Clinic – Helios Clinic,
Aukammallee 33, Wiesbaden D 65191, Germany
e-mail: Risikomanagement.Merkle@hotmail.de

© Springer-Verlag Berlin Heidelberg 2016
W. Merkle (ed.), *Risk Management in Medicine*, DOI 10.1007/978-3-662-47407-5_1

Both diagnostic and therapeutic procedures are focused when discussing failure management. Therefore not only surgical disciplines but also so-called conservative disciplines are involved.

In Germany we have the institution of so-called medical expert commissions regarding every single discipline to decide about correct or incorrect procedures done in case a patient might have the opinion something went wrong during his medical treatment.

This institution is a specific German way of dealing with malpractice but has many advantages – it is independent, objective, and broadly accepted by doctors, patients, lawyers, and insurance companies – and furthermore it avoids the official way to court. In case somebody does not accept the decision of this expert commission, he/she is free to go to court. However, approximately 97 % of expert decisions are confirmed by court which shows the high professionalism of the specific German way to deal with suspected malpractice. Details are presented in Chap. 2.

The most important principle of successful risk management is called "Kaizen."

This Japanese word means: thank you for learning from you (from your mistake).

The acceptance of this principle should come first in medicine all over the world.

Other businesses are far more developed in this important tool or risk management.

Aviation business works as THE key developer.

Everything started with the announcement of all failures that have occurred during a flight – free of punishment.

Thus repeated, that means principle failures were quickly detected and could be solved. This gave the chance of fast improvement in flying safety.

Furthermore the experience of a single airline was communicated openly, thus all other airlines could learn a parallel. The overall flying risks were reduced and meanwhile flying has proved to be much safer than other forms of transportation.

The culture of blame – current status in medicine – hinders a fast improvement in avoiding failure.

Eventually there are psychological causes, too, when being of the opinion: "I'm a doctor, I do all my procedures correctly."

This ethos is nothing more than claim, but not reality.

1.2   First Steps of Failure Theory

During the 1960, Motorola started with the systematic analysis of failures that occurred. Shortly after the PCDA cyclus was developed followed by the 6-Sigma strategy the first perception was: we ALL make mistakes.

In medicine, the Harvard Medical School showed impressively that 3 % of medical procedures were performed incorrectly (www.hms.harvard.edu). Well, this huge amount of failures does mean death cases or severe problems – most mistakes are harmless, but not to forget – also death cases are included.

Of course the main focus on strategies reducing failures is on harmful mistakes.

The first step is called Failure Analysis.

It is constructed of product quality together with structure quality and process quality.

It depends on competence in basic knowledge, methods, and social behavior.

In the field of medicine this means

- Product quality: operation successful?
- Structure quality: modern hospital with modern equipment; well-trained and educated staff working with the current knowledge in their field?
- Process quality: e.g., correct timing and following of the different steps of an OR procedure (lean management)?

Competence means

- In knowledge: Are the involved doctor and staff well educated for this specific case or is there a colleague (in another hospital) better qualified for this patient?
- In methods: do, e.g., the surgeons govern all kinds of procedures for this specific case, thus the patient has the chance to make a free

decision? For example, in hernia surgery, does the surgeon know to operate conventionally with the Shouldice procedure, Lichtenstein net, or laparoscopically, etc.

- In social behavior: reducing fear, explaining individually what is planned, accepting patient's decision, accepting partnership between patient and doctor, etc.

Important to know – lacking social competence will likely lead to court if something goes wrong whereas patients might otherwise accept a minor mistake if the doctor speaks frankly about what's going wrong and shows his/her personal concern and apologizes to the patient and family members.

On the other hand, arrogance is the "easiest" way to court and is to be blamed.

1.3   Human Factor

There are two contradictive statements:

- Humans are able to think complex, so although with a limited data basis correct decisions can be made.
- Humans are emotionally driven, so failures in their doing are imminent: praise improves correct outcome; being critical reduces success.

In summary humans are better than machines when complex processes and procedures like operations have to be performed.

Thus standardization including guidelines is helpful but should never press someone into a rigid corset as humans are principally individuals (Perabo 2012).

Meanwhile in Germany even the high court has accepted that "guidelines guide," but they are not laws which have to be strictly followed (Chap. 15).

Consequently failure analysis, reduction by PDCA, and risk management are the way to go. To shorten learning process and avoid a long learning curve medicine should learn from parallel disciplines and adopt experience.

The most appropriate technique to install is the FMEA (Chap. 11) (Failure Mode and Effects Analysis).

Another analogue in dealing with complex procedures under limited data basis and also human driven is aviation business.

The parallels are impressive:

- Complex technique
- High stress level
- Many things to do parallelly in very short time
- Working against biorhythm (e.g., during the night)
- Limited resources
- Limited personnel

However, we all are used to safe journeys by plane, almost not even thinking about the inherent problems of going into the air.

How could this occur?

The answer is more or less simple – consequent risk management.

Risk management in medicine is lacking, as the following tables show:

Differences between medicine and airlines:
Airlines

- Strict failure management
- Consequent use of checklists
- Teamwork with flat hierarchy
- Open dealing with conflicts
- Observing soft skills
- Regular training in simulator
- Consequent support of zero-failure strategy by management (including financial support)
- SAFETY IS THE MAIN CONCERN

Medicine

- No risk management
- Culture of blame
- No support by management
- Under-refunding
- Reduction of personnel
- Disregarding soft skills
- COST REDUCTION is the main concern

Therefore the president of the German "Landesärztekammer Hessen" pointed out,

"Health policy and public insurance companies were looking more for cost reduction instead of improving curative elements" (Hess. Ärztebl. 8/2011, pp 468–69).

Although this is a German statement, more or less it is common all over the world.

However, in the medical business meanwhile doctors found out that it pays to learn from the flight crew (*J. Urology* 2011:185:1177–78). The reason is clear – the main risk for fatal outcome as well in airline business as in medicine is a combination of failures in communication and rigid hierarchy.

For example, "the fundamental cause of catastrophes (total loss) was not ice, snow, fog or empty fuel tanks but hierarchy" (*J. Urol.* 2011). Consequently this finding is the question: "How to turn a team of experts into an expert medical team?" (Burke et al. 2004). This is the question for CRM (Crew Resource Management).

CRM in medicine is more or less unknown although teamwork is routine but not professionally learned.

The main topics of CRM are

- Briefing before operation start – including everybody
- Explaining expected critical points of the operation
- Discussion about potential risk of the individual patient
- Freedom for everybody to show concerns
- Short briefing report in patient's file

For details, see Chap. 14.

Additionally in case the operation reaches a critical point, TTO (Team Time-Out) is a successful tool to reduce the risk of the situation. Also here, there is no hierarchy. Everybody in the team shall contribute.

There are two further aspects to know – very human in its kind.

Night shift work is a safety risk for doctors' own health – leading to diabetes, heart attacks, discomfort of the GI system, and (!) increased risk for accidents (e.g., when driving back home) (Straif et al. 2007).

By chronoadopted work shift this inherent problem can be reduced (Straif et al. 2007).

Furthermore – doctors who are blamed by patients show increased levels of depression and of commiting suicide (Bourne et al. 2015). Therefore it is very wise to reduce any failures which can be followed by blaming and lawsuit.

Thus, the human factor problem affects not only patients but also the staff. This at least should be the most important cause accepting risk management thus reducing the very own risk of working at a hospital.

1.4 Methods

Communication first!

Yes, this is correct, more or less. While a targeted communication process improves problem solving, overboarding communication will lead to even more failures.

Why?

The OTAS study (Chap. 10) clearly pointed out that unnecessary communication risked concentration of the surgeon as well as of the team thus increasing failure level. Details will be shown in Chap. 10.

On the other hand, if communication is avoided, important information might be lacking.

In aviation business this is well known.

Therefore, "empower lower-ranking crew members to voice their concerns in a respectful but assertive manner. Teach higher-ranking members to listen to the crew and view questions as signs of honest concern for clarification but not as insubordination or doubts about the leader's ability" (*J. Urol.* 2011).

1.5 Use of Checklists

In principle checklists are helpful tools to avoid overlooking important things to do. However, there is not one single type of checklist but as many checklists as there are hospitals.

What is appropriate for, e.g., the Vanderbilt University Hospital will definitely not fit for a small clinic in the Australian Outback and vice versa.

Thus it is mandatory that each hospital founds a work group to make an individual checklist of this specific hospital. However there are principal checklists on the market assisting and tailoring such a list for each individual clinic. How to use checklists effectively can be found in the chapter on TTO.

Furthermore checklists cannot avoid all major failures.

There are specific risks from economy.

For example, it is simple to prove whether OR instruments are complete prior to or after an operation.

But a checklist cannot teach about the quality of the instruments. In the online press service of a German newspaper it was reported that most OR instruments are produced in Sialkot, Pakistan, independent of which brand name is printed on the instrument itself.

Most of these instruments are good quality, however a certain number are of minor quality although they look analog – the surgeon cannot find this out prior to use.

And one can imagine which might be the fatal consequences of a broken instrument, etc.

There is only one solution – buying instruments by the administration must be triggered mostly by quality instead of price – especially because many of the low budget instruments are produced by children. This must be avoided.

A specific technical risk is found in the hospital IT.

This is twofold – first using computer programs for administration work and storing patients' data. The inherent problems of this field are similar to routine application in other businesses, e.g., current version of software, proper and actual hardware, maintenance, and regular teaching of staff using those programs. Most people are more or less familiar with this problem field.

Second – and this is overlooked and not correctly appreciated – we have to face cyber criminality also using IT technology in hospitals. Many hospitals do not work with cryptic programs and firewalls although dealing with sensitive data is the key process in hospitals – personal data of patients including their health status are sensitive – for example, the status of Steve Jobs' disease was of importance for Apple Industries. Although most data were public by press and TV, some weren't, although they were noticed in the hospital file. In case these secret data would have been public no one can imagine what the consequences would have been.

Not everybody is so prominent, but a patient's personal health record should be kept private.

Thus not even a hacker should have access to the hospital's computer files.

And not to forget – data security is enforced by law.

Nevertheless the following examples show impressively that many hospitals have an open flank.

1.6 Problems of Technical Failures

There are not only problems imminent of medical instruments but also by maintenance process. Regular check of all instruments especially when the procedure is complex, e.g., daVinci OR robot or laparoscopic devices, is mandatory. Never should this be neglected although it costs money.

Consequent use of checklists (provided by the manufacturer) avoids nonfunctioning medical devices when they are used before starting the operation – comparable to the routine check of an aircraft prior to boarding of passengers.

1.6.1 Examples of IT-Specific Risks

Many processes are steered by DICOM interfaces like MRI or CT scanners using Windows software. Updates of Windows software come regularly to close unsafe program tools. Thus everything seems safe – but not in hospitals. By law hospital software has to be certified. This certification needs time – and every single update has to be certified by its own. Thus updates come regularly – certification not. Therefore hospital software is permanently relatively old, and underfunding of public hospitals worsens this additionally because updating and certification costs money.

The second problem is found in the speed of hardware development. Renewals cost additional money.

The consequence is an open flank in IT security because hospitals tend to give priority to medical devices more if money is short.

Criminals take their chance to enter the hospital IT by, e.g., Trojan horses and ransom ware. In Australia hackers encoded the software and extorted money (www.abc.net.au).

Another example from Germany: Back-up CDs were transported in a suitcase by a staff member. He wanted to smoke, and during this period the suitcase was not properly watched. Returning from his cigarette break he missed his suitcase – it was never found (www.welt.de).

The next example happened in Massachusetts. A laptop with miserable encrypting programming was lost. It contained 3500 personal patients' files. The fee by the Department of Health and Human Services reached the sum of $1.5 million (www.threatpost.com).

(These examples were provided by Patrick Helmig, Security by Culture, Wiesbaden, Germany.)

Additionally, complex medical techniques including IT techniques borrow principle problems by their own:

- Problem of flashback: malfunctioning software might generate failures in a principally properly working machine after it's connected to the hospital's IT system (e.g., by Trojan horses, worms, virus, etc.).
- Correct transmission of data: are all necessary data in the doctor's hand? And just in time?
- Timely components: the more components between sender and receiver of information, the longer the way, thus more time consumed.
- Interpretation: due to the huge amount of data available which nobody can process completely, programs assist to reduce this data tsunami. However, by this processing, important

data might be missing thereafter because the filter was not properly adjusted.

These complex themes can be found in the international norm (IEC 80001–1). It is recommended to read it carefully and draw all necessary consequences.

Although this is a technical field *sui generis* all doctors must know about it, because medical diagnosis and treatment as well as decision-making are influenced today by IT and technique.

The hospital administration has to make every effort to reduce these risks close to zero.

1.7 The Zero-Failure Strategy

1.7.1 Doing It Right the First Time!

This motto describes shortly the principle of failure and quality management respectively.

Plan – Do – Check – Act is implemented into a circle (Fig. 1.1), which is also known as 6–sigma process.

More or less this process deals with analysis of the entire work done, whether it fits with the rules or shows deviations which have to be corrected. After correction the result has to be proven in the mirror of rules.

Thus in many single and short acts failures will be reduced. But this has to be done permanently.

Of course improvement of quality and reduction of risks cost money, time, and personnel. On the other side it reduced total costs through reduction of costs to solve a failure.

It is mandatory not to invent the wheel again but to optimize current processes.

Analogues to the aviation business are obvious. Optimizing flight routes save kerosene and reduce the risk of total loss, etc.

In the same manner optimizing in medicine reduces bringing an action against the hospital or doctor which would cost reputation and money too – not to forget avoiding human sorrow.

Fig. 1.1 DMAIC Cyclus

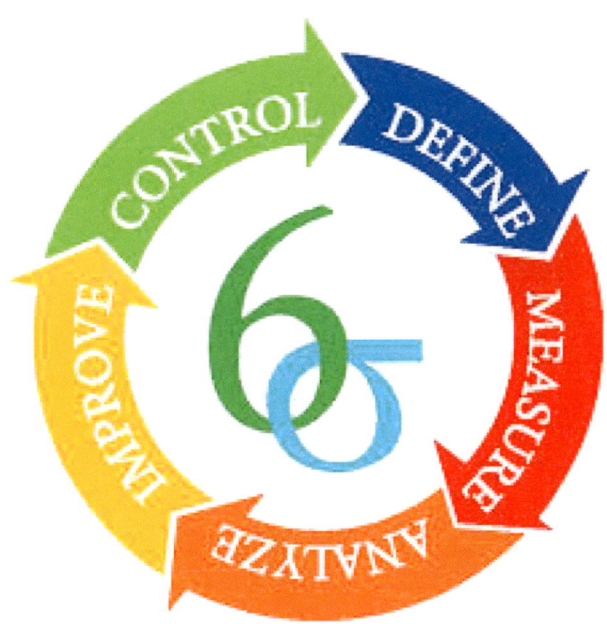

1.8   Problems with Saving Money

- Overaged equipment (=reduced quality, more often repair)
- Reduced personnel
- Minor educated personnel
- Reduced quality of buildings
- Unproven modernization

This list contains important problems following cost reduction process. They all have in common the increased risk of breakdowns and cancellation which immediately reduces income and directly increases costs.

Overaged equipment is followed by exhaustion of material which causes increased costs for maintenance and repair, thus the amount of repair exceeds the price of new equipment.

This is the standpoint of business administration, but even more important is the standpoint of medical safety. Overaged equipment increases the risk for being liable for failures – this is the clear standpoint of the German High Court.

The individual doctor has to be fit in the current techniques of his specialty – which includes the use of modern material and techniques.

In case this would not be provided by the hospital he has to transfer his patient to a better-equipped hospital to protect him from possible failures!

1.8.1   Shortage of Personnel

In a current study of three American hospitals (UCLA, Mayo-Clinic, Duke University) their pooled data clearly demonstrated that reducing staff members will be followed by increased mortality of patients – if one single nurse is missing on a ward the mortality increases 2.7 % in total. If the main causes for death are isolated mortality increases by 5 % – these data are significant (Needleman et al. 2011)!

Cahill et al. (2011) wrote, "Shockingly the authors estimated that the risk of death increased by 2 % for each below-target shift and 4 % for each high-turnover shift experienced by a given patient."

The lack of nurses is well known – patients have to pay this with their lives.

It is the decision of a society how much saved money a human life is worth!

Shortage of personnel is an organization deficit of the hospital administration.

1.8.2 Minor Qualification

Well-educated and trained personnel are expensive due to high(er) payment. Therefore it seems attractive to reduce hospital costs by taking lower-qualified personnel. On the other hand, risk of overlooked patient problems will follow – with all consequences.

Whether SOPs might help solve this gap remains unclear. It will be doubtful whether a court would accept a SOP as substitution of lacking qualified personnel in the case of an accident or medical failure.

1.8.3 Quality of Buildings

The main risk of older hospital buildings is lack of proper hygiene.

MRSA and ESBL can be prevented partly by optimizing buildings and furniture.

Furthermore, old buildings with long corridors waste (staff) time, thus money.

1.8.4 Unproven Modernization

"New and modern" are not strictly synonyms for "good and correct."

Normally, a new product – e.g., a new laparoscopic instrument – should be proven in a large check procedure. However due to high costs of this procedure often a small series of hospitals and patients respectively must be enough before this new product will be brought to market.

This is like "flying on (almost) untested wings."

And the indication for such a new procedure might be stressed and widened charging the patient with the unknown risk.

An example is the new pelvic floor meshes in Gynecology and Urology. The FDA statement is clear: "POP can be treated successfully without mesh thus avoiding the risk of mesh-related complications."

Other procedures do not stand the test of time. Therefore before a new method should be implemented in a hospital, correct testing is mandatory.

Patients do know about these specific risks of hurrying when a new procedure is decided.

Furthermore, the more economic aspects lead the hospital management, the more patients become distrustful.

Additionally due to economic aspects, the patient will be divided in different organs. So billing is easier; the amount of earned money for the hospital can be "optimized" (=increased). Doing this will be followed by overlooking important information. The procedures' risk level will rise.

To reduce interruption and save money by avoiding idleness, a balance score card is helpful. Four perspectives are under parallel view: customer/patient – finance – process – development. This multidimensional model can be optimized increasing the efficiency of the OR in total.

There is a further risk – raisin picking. In times in which some procedures/operations are highly priced, some are almost neglected under the aspect of earning money (e.g., psychosomatic medicine, etc.) Unethical decision-making might occur to stretch the indications for "valuable" operations – eventually not correctly respecting patients' needs and interests.

More or less healing of a disease mutates to just a repair.

But the guarantee for a repair is much higher than for curing a disease. Therefore this fatal direction of medicine must be avoided.

Standardization is another source for failures and risks.

Sure, most procedures can be optimized by accepting standards.

But only the individual procedures give the spice of well-being. Therefore it is current German law that standards are important helpful tools for the individual but they are nothing more; they are just guidelines, which can help, e.g., when the procedure is rare or relatively new.

1.9 Risk by Organization of Work

Bus drivers, pilots, and other personnel in transportation services have to obey strict working hours and are strict about breaking these rules.

This is absolutely mandatory and correct because overtiredness will lead to failures and fatal accidents. Even on long-distance flights there is an additional pilot resting to replace the pilot flying after several hours in charge.

In the field of medicine those strict rules are more or less unknown.

In Europe it was necessary to bring these rules to the European High Court, which decided – of course – for a strict break schedule especially after night shifts and weekend shifts. However the shortage of available doctors in some fields and/or regions led to weakening these rules unfortunately.

The Association of Anaesthetics of Great Britain published the results of a study in 2005 which shows evidently the consequences of over-extended working hours: The coordination of hand to eye worsens significantly – especially important in surgical disciplines.

Since 2003 the "effect of sleep deprivation on performance of simulated laparoscopic surgical skills" is well known (Eastridge et al. 2003). Overtiredness was followed by a significant amount of technical failures depending on the length of this period of sleep deprivation. It is only a question of time when a fatal failure will definitely occur!

The longer the work shift, the more often are medical errors. After a 17 h shift the work performance was comparable to blood alcohol level of 0.5‰. After 24 h this worsens to an equivalent of 100 g alcohol (this is about one bottle of red wine!).

Furthermore, the more long shifts happen, the more is the strain of staff. In the Whitehall Study II it was demonstrated that the next consequence is mental depression and increased amount of heart attacks (Marmot et al., 1991; Virtanen et al. 2010) as well as exhaustion (Gaba and Howard 2002).

All these procedures are in conflict with current rules. The fast idea to organize the work in three different shifts of 8 h is not unproblematic. Regular shifts working against the biological rhythm of a body will sooner or later lead to health problems and increased failure rates (v. Manteuffel 2011). Furthermore, a brand new Chinese meta-analysis reviewing more than 226,000 participants (!) pointed out clearly that the risk to develop diabetes significantly increased in shift working. The highest risk level was measured in rotating shift models between early, late, and night shifts (*Occup Environ Med.* 2014 doi:10.1136/oemed-2014-102150).

Regular shift work suffers from systemic failures of incomplete information to the following shift members. Written information might prevent this, but the personal impression of an experienced nurse or doctor cannot be replaced by bureaucracy. Therefore it remains mandatory to train personnel in these pitfalls to be aware of handing over patients from shift staff to shift staff.

Thus there is no simple solution except to have enough personnel to protect the patients and the staff members as well.

This obviously costs money. In the aviation business this is not the point of discussion – safety is the primary concern even if it costs money.

Unfortunately in the medical business this kind of safety concern is not present although it should be. This will definitely cost lives.

1.10 Mobbing

Even when work organization and all circumstances are optimal, problems can occur.

Cause can be problems between people. Mobbing meanwhile is a well-known phenomenon. It costs work power and reduces the ROI (return on investment).

And it is a main source for failures.

The mobbing victim is excluded from information thus it works suboptimally which – and this is important – will do harm to patients.

Furthermore, the closer a work process is, the more bossing can occur (Litzcke and Schuh 2007) because

In principle all people are susceptible to psychological influences – also for the negative ones.

The well-known pyramid of Maslow and Herzberg (Fig. 1.2) demonstrates the background. Self-realization is on top of motivation causes.

Fig. 1.2 Maslow'
pyramide

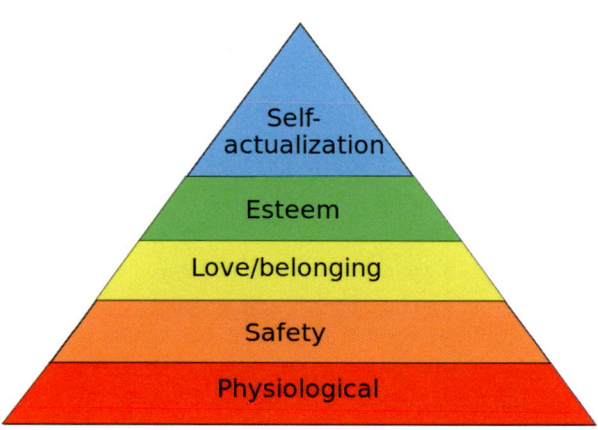

Thus in case this is disturbed by the opposite partner it is in the foreseeable future that failures and low work performance will follow.

1.11 Peer Review

Insiders know where there could be problems, thus they can directly look at these points.

PR detects lack in interdisciplinary teamwork, deciding for the correct indications, coordination, and correct file management.

Therefore it is – especially with doctors – widely accepted. PR can detect typical medicine failures which can be overcome by the doctors themselves. Thus the learning effect is very high. Details can be found in Chap. 13.

1.12 LASA

Look alike sound alike. This is a typical problem in medications.

Thus similar brand names can be mixed up. But also dosages might be confused.

Examples are Lasix – Losec; Cefuroxim – Cefotaxim, etc.

And in a hectic atmosphere easily µg and mg can be mixed up. The consequences can be fatal.

How to solve this problem? When writing in block letters the staff member's eye will reduce its speed thus reading slowly thus correctly, e.g., CALCium – COTRim forte, etc. And the doctor's handwriting problem is solved additionally, too.

Hearing failures can be avoided by repeating what was heard, thus the one talking has the chance to correct the wrong hearing. Furthermore writing down what was heard and countersigning it is also a way to increase safety.

Meanwhile there is some software available when ordering some medication, the so-called computerized provider order entry (DÄB 2011, 36 Bl 570–73).

1.13 Self-Estimation

In cases the self-estimation of the very own capability can be a cause for failures when the estimation is incorrect.

A questionnaire was given to pilots and doctors (cockpit/flight/OR management attitudes questionnaire) and filled. The result is amazing.

1. "Tiredness does not reduce capability significantly."
   Pilots agreed in 26 % whereas surgeons agreed in 70 %; they estimated their capability to be sufficient although they were tired.
2. "Avoiding a strict hierarchy is mandatory."
   Pilots agreed in an impressive 97 % whereas surgeons accept this statement only in 55 %; but the staff or an ICU agreed similar to the pilots in 94 %.
3. "We do perform teamwork."
   Surgeons believe that they are part of a team in 73 %. Nurses believe this in only 35–38 %.

Additionally the staff members of an ICU believe, "I do not make mistakes."

The consequence of these different self-estimations is: Pilots are aware of a principle problem of self-estimation and accept that they can make mistakes. This attitude protects against failures. On the other hand, overconfidence of doctors causes overlooking of problems and neglecting their own risk to make mistakes, thus failures cannot be prevented.

The culture of blame in many hospitals is an additional cause why doctors act as if they are blameless.

The solution of this conflict can be found in accepting their own faulty work and the principles and acceptance to learn from failures. Learning from others is also an important tool (Sexton et al. 2000; see Chap. 4).

1.14 Guidelines

Guidelines at first glance seem to be a simple and effective solution as a risk management tool.

But it is mandatory to know that guidelines are not strictly enforced laws but information guiding a doctor through the jungle of differential diagnosis and the desert of different durative procedures. The German High Court has clearly pointed out this important statement for over 40 years. The cause can easily be understood: human beings and their diseases are absolutely individual, thus a guideline as law can never cope with every single case, thus guidelines shall assist but give the doctor the freedom to decide individually in the individual patient's case.

How strict enforcement of "guidelines" can end is shown in Chap. 5 where it is demonstrated why an Airbus A 340–600 ran against a wall. The medical explanation can be found with Perabo (2012).

1.15 Ways to Solve the Problem(s)

In many hospitals it is absolutely mandatory for new strategies to emerge.

The culture of blame must be given up, living CIRS and FMEA must be installed – and be integrated in daily practice.

A culture of trust must be brought to life. KAIZEN is the target to find – in all management levels.

Kaizen is Japanese. It means: Thank you that I was permitted to learn from your faults.

Flat hierarchy and the acceptance of teamwork where everybody has to contribute without undermining authority are important tools as well as the principal acceptance of the very own failures made.

Resources of personnel and money will be paid back by a more successful medicine reducing failure costs.

The risk management techniques described in this textbook will contribute to a positive culture of failure management. The high rate of principal failures in medicine which currently reaches approximately 3 % (Harvard Study) will be reduced. Medicine will reach similar safety like the aviation business achieved within the last 50 years coming down from a risky transportation system to a safe means of mass transport.

1.16 Zero-Failure Strategy

It is the final target.

An interesting tool on this way of improvement can be found in standardization. The ISO 9001 was developed as industrial standard; meanwhile the ISO 15224 was established which is adopted for health care providers. *Details are found in* Chap. 21.

But it must be pointed out clearly:

The main risk in medicine is the gap between safety and earning money.

Society has to give strict regulations where the borderline is found between increasing the ROI of a hospital and spending money for improvement of a patient's safety.

This is a political process to be performed in advance – not after a patient's injury has happened due to saving money for an anonymous shareholder.

It will be thrilling to find out how much medicine safety and safe lives are worth to society.

Literature

17: Apps im Gesundheitswesen. www.springermedizin. de/keine-chance-dem-kunstfehler/37546.html

Bourne T, Wynants L, Peters M, Audenhove CV, Timmerman D, Calster BV, Jalmbrant M (2015) The impact of complaints procedures on the welfare, health and clinical practise of 7926 doctors in the UK: a cross-sectional survey Press Release. BMJ Open 5:e006687. doi:10.1136/bmjopen-2014-006687

Burke et al (2004) Qual Saf Health Care 13(Suppl):196

Cahill M, Kevin W, Michael Y (2011) More nurses means fewer inpatient deaths. Neurosurgery 69(4):N15–N16. doi:10.1227/01.neu.0000405593.93707.88

DÄB 2011, 36, B1570–73

Eastridge BJ, Hamilton EC, O'Keefe GE, Rege RV, Valentine RJ, Jones DJ, Tesfay S, Thal ER (2003) Effect of sleep deprivation on the performance of simulated laparoscopic surgical skill. Am J Surg 186(2):169–174

Gaba D, Howard SK (2002) Patient safety: fatigue among clinicians and the safety of patients. N Engl J Med 347(16):1249–1255

Gerstenkorn (2012) Auch Chirurgen brauchen Pausen. OP-Impuls 2:17–18

Klotz T (2012) Priorisierung in der medizin. In: Rübben H, Otto T (ed)Colloquium urologie. pp 3–13

Litzcke S, Schuh H (2007) Stress, mobbing und burn-out am arbeitsplatz, 4th edn. Springer, Heidelberg

Manteuffel LV (2011) DÄB, 50, C2 234–35

Marmot MG, Smith GD, Stansfeld S, Patel C, North F, Head J, White I, Brunner E, Feeney A (1991) Health inequalities among British civil servants: the Whitehall II study. Lancet 337(8754):1387–1393

Merkle W (2002) Komplikationen nach TVT-plastik. In: Steffens J, Langen PH (eds) Komplikationen in der urologie. Steinkopff, Darmstadt, pp 135–137

Needleman J et al (2011) N Engl J Med 364:1037–1045

Perabo (2012) Plenum II, DGU. Leipzig

Sexton JB et al (2000) Error, stress and teamwork in medicine and aviation: cross sectional surveys. BMJ 320:745–749

Straif K et al (2007) Lancet Oncol 8(12):1065–1066. In: www.medscapemedizin.de/artikelansicht/4903259

Stredele R et al (2012) DGU, Abstract. p 16.6

Virtanen M, Kivimäki M et al (2010) Work disability following major organisational change: the Whitehall II study. J Epidemiol Community Health 64:461–464. doi:10.1136/jech.2009.095158

Current View of German Authorities (State Chamber of Physicians)

Roland H. Kaiser

Abstract

There is a specific German way dealing with malpractice, the so-called Gutachterkommission. It enables discussing the case without going to court although medical experts are taking care for each case. Thus, acceptance from both sides is high. The rate of accepted malpractice is around one third of all cases. This rate is constant over the last decade.

The chapter will point out this successful way.

2.1 Assessment and Conciliation Boards of the State Chambers of Physicians

2.1.1 Gutachter- und Schlichtungsstellen der Ärztekammern – GUS[1]

Assessment and conciliation boards of medical chambers were established in 1975. Some state chambers (e.g. Hessen) operate these facilities independently, and others cooperate within the structure of a "conciliation body for medical malpractice litigation, arbitration and mediation of the Northern German chambers of physicians"

(Bundesärztekammer 2015a). All these expert and mediation boards cooperate and participate in a yearly national conference. All expert and mediation boards operate according to a similar basic principle of methodology, an example of which used by Hessen is described below.

Data of all national GUS boards have been recorded since 1979, and a "Medical Error Reporting System" (MERS) was established in 2006 for compiling and publishing nationwide statistics. This data is freely accessible to the public via the website of the National Medical Chamber (Bundesärztekammer 2015b).

The total number of applications submitted to evaluation boards has slightly risen from 10,280 in 2006 to 12,173 in 2013. In 2013, 7.922 decisions were taken which represented 66 % of all applications. 23.5 % of these were deemed as damages with causal links to a medical malpractice and/or a lack of clarification, and 4.8 % were assessed as damages without causal links. In 71.7 % of decisions, no wrongful conduct was found. Application for assessment of possibly incorrect treatment in

---

[1] This is a conciliation board of the chamber of physicians dealing with law suit not handled by official courts.

R.H. Kaiser, MD
Landesärztekammer Hessen,
Im Vogelsgesang 3, Frankfurt 60488, Germany
e-mail: roland.kaiser@laekh.de

© Springer-Verlag Berlin Heidelberg 2016
W. Merkle (ed.), *Risk Management in Medicine*, DOI 10.1007/978-3-662-47407-5_2

both hospitals and private practices was predominantly for the medical areas of surgery, emergency surgery and orthopaedics with treated diagnoses of coxarthrosis and gonarthrosis.

The assessment and conciliation board of the chamber in Hessen (Gutachter- und Schlichtungsstelle der Landesärztekammer Hessen) was founded in 1978 and is headed by Dr. Katharina Deppert (presiding judge at the BGH, emeritus). It is independent not bound by any instructions (Landesärztekammer 2015). Upon an application by a patient or a physician, the board provides a nonjudicial dispute settlement scheme with the goal of defining whether an avoidable treatment mistake with a resulting injury has been committed. Requests for such investigations are mostly made by patient, rarely physicians.

2.1.2 Definition of Medical Malpractice

In accordance with GUS standards, a diagnostic or medical procedure is termed a medical malpractice or insufficient treatment if:

- The procedure or intervention was not medically indicated.
- Not all due diligence according to the latest findings of the medical sciences and clinical practice was objectively shown or it remained largely unaddressed.
- There is failure to intervene according to the measure of medical grounds.

An injurious treatment (iatrogenic harm) is defined as the "general term for all injuries and damage to health which did not result from immanent complications, but originated in preventable treatment errors or through inevitable treatment-immanent effects".

The assessment and conciliation board does not act if any legal procedures concerning a putative treatment mistake have already been initiated, or a court rule has been issued.

The involvement of the conciliation board is free of charge for both patients and physicians. The costs incurred are paid for by the chamber, with liability insurers providing a set amount via a defined contribution scheme. The physician's liability insurer is informed by the physician or the board. The conciliation board requests the patient's medical files and appoints an independent expert consultant. The choice of expert consultant can be contested within 3 weeks of the consultant's nomination. The conciliation board issues the consultant's independently formed appraisal, in the form of an evaluation, to all parties involved. The board procedure is completed upon the issue of a written reasoned commission decision to all parties. An involvement of the conciliation board does not exclude the possibility of subsequent legal action. In almost all cases, though, legal procedures reconfirmed the decision of the commission of the conciliation board – in the past, only 3 % of legal complaints brought to action rendered a deviating decision.

2.1.3 Advantages of the GUS Procedure Compared to Judicial Court Proceedings

The most important advantages for a patient injured by a putative treatment mistake are:

(a) The application for appraisal and the board procedure are free of charge.
(b) The GUS procedure is more time-effective and with a more immediate response than judicial court proceedings.
(c) There is high propensity of liability insurers to accept the board's decision and subsequent willingness to pay compensation fees without initiating further legal charges. Another advantage not to be underestimated is the psychological aspect – the board procedure has shown to be less emotionally impacted for an applicant than judicial court proceedings. Altogether, the work of the assessment and conciliation boards is held in high esteem by both physicians and liability insurers. Physicians who are accused of putative treatment mistakes profit from the elimination drawn-out legal battles and confrontational disputes with their insurers.

The expert consultants' appraisals requested by the board commissions act as important sources of information for the analysis of treatment errors and systematically prevent future mistakes, functioning comparably to a CIRS procedure.

In 2013, the conciliation board received 902 new applications for assessment. 887 of those were completed, 498 with reasoned commission decisions. 122 of these cases (24.5 %) were ruled as factual treatment mistakes responsible for the assessed injury, and in 372 (74.5 %) cases, no treatment mistakes were confirmed.

2.1.4 Differentiation of Various Areas of Medicine, Indications and Separate Sectors of Health Care

Sixty-one percent of all physicians affected by board procedures were resident doctors at hospitals and 39 % were in private practice. 50 % of all hospital cases and 44 % of cases in ambulant care evaluated were in the medical fields of visceral surgery/orthopaedics/trauma surgery, but it nevertheless should not be inferred that treatment mistakes occur far more often in surgery than in internal medicine. Surgical procedures often provide more conspicuous, more strictly defined and detailed documentation to be used for assessment. Patients often have substantial but often not realistic expectations concerning the result or success of an operation/surgical procedure. If the hoped-for result is not achieved (e.g. a frequent occasion with indications such as coxarthrosis or gonarthrosis) or complications occur, the patient is more likely to suspect a complication resulting from malpractice. This is less likely to occur with an unfavourable development of an internal medicine treating long-term condition. Hence, it is not surprising that most applications for the investigation of treatment mistakes are concerning damages resulting from surgery. As a general rule, treatment mistakes and their cause for resulting injuries are easier to detect and prove by an expert, when they occur in surgical or other invasive diagnostical procedures unlike those

suspected or committed in conservative therapies. Treatment mistakes in the fields of psychiatry and psychotherapy, despite the comparably higher numbers of patient contacts, are rarely subject of an assessment.

Therefore, the primary focus of all risk management schemes for hospitals and private practices is the areas involving surgical measurements. But, after the implementation of measures in these areas, it is imperative that the so-called conservative fields of medicine have to be included; the incorrect administration of medication is a frequent mistake committed, often with fatal results. Regarding all decisions issued by the board, the rate of 20–25 % of cases determined treatment mistakes is remarkably constant (2008, 22 %; 2011, 24 %; 2012, 23 %; 2013, 24.5 %), a number which is consistent with the national statistical rate.

2.2 Mistakes Committed in Daily Medical Practice and Patient Rights from the Vantage of German State Chambers of Physicians

2.2.1 Introduction

"Primum nil (non) nocere". The historical development of the patient-physician relationship to the decentralized, hi-tech, complex and specialized medical care of today has resulted in a number of additional new risks and potential complications. Besides basic problems caused by medical progress, these include technical defects, adverse drug reactions, miscommunications and spectacular mix-ups in large health institutions. The most effective action for treatment error prevention and reduction in modern medicine may be an improved and more critical indication for all potentially harmful medical measurements. Mistakes are not entirely avoidable; therefore, early detection is vital to reduce or prevent damages and to learn to avoid recurrences of similar errors out of pure self-interest for the medical field.

The current social perception of errors and risks and the discussion of patient safety and patient rights are not just results of a modernized, technically-scientifically characterized medicine but are potentially an expression of the formal-juristic and economical culture predominant in Western industrial nations today. Physicians are "service providers" and patients are "customers or case figures" and components of a "case mix". Complications are the basis for civil damage claims, lack of documentation results in reversal of the burden of proof, etc. The often undifferentiated, sensationalized reporting on spectacular "medical malpractices" evokes guaranteed high ratings for today's printed press and increasingly electronic mass media. This does not facilitate the handling and prevention of errors in patient care for physicians or medical associations. Experience has shown that mistakes occur primarily when humans act under high pressure and/or time limitations. As the 108th Deutsche Ärztetag (108th German Medical Assembly) accurately pointed out in 2005: "Cost pressure and competition result in undifferentiated savings, resulting in jeopardizing the standards of patient care. A higher amount of patients are cared for by fewer health care providers using increasingly complex diagnosis and treatment methods in ever decreasing time periods. A new demand for the development of error prevention strategies in clinics and private practices is needed to adapt to these changing conditions" (Deutscher Ärztetag 2005).

Those who know more and are better educated make less mistakes! The regional chambers have therefore been offering a wide variety of training measures and information seminars on error prevention and risk management for both physician members as well as medical assistants.

In 8–12 % of patients admitted to a hospital in EU member states, a severe incident during a medical treatment or intervention occurred (TNS Opinion & Social 2010). The European Centre for Prevention and Control (ECDC) estimated that 5 % of hospital patients develop HCAIs (health-care-associated infections) leading to 37,000 deaths annually (Scheppokat 2009). A survey of various studies mainly from Switzerland showed that 3–4 % of patients treated in hospitals suffer health damages resulting from treatment

(Scheppokat and Neu 2007). Approximately one fourth of these damages were caused by treatment mistakes.

From 2001, a publication by the American Institute of Medicine (Kohn et al. 2000) called "To Err is Human" triggered intensive discussions in Germany on errors committed by physicians and the resulting damages in patients. In September/October 2009, a study commissioned by the EU commission was conducted using 26,663 personal interviews to ensure a representative sample of EU citizens aged 15 and over from 27 member states.

Topics of the survey were these citizens' views on patient safety and quality of medical care. Interesting results of the study (TNS Opinion & Social 2010) included:

- 50 % of respondents (EU), 31 % of Germans (D) but only 19 % of Austrians (AT) considered it likely that patients could suffer from a treatment-related damage resulting from an inpatient or outpatient treatment in their respective country. (Austrian results are used for comparison as they represented the lowest expected values of all EU countries, while its health-care system shares many common elements with the German system.) 46 % (EU), 65 % (D) and 79 % (AT) considered the occurrence of a treatment-related damage unlikely.
- 46 % of EU citizens, 29 % of Germans and 24 % of Austrians considered damages occurring from nonhospital care provided by a general physician or pharmacist as probable, and 49 % (EU), 66 % (D) and 73 % (AT) deemed them unlikely.
- 25 % of EU citizens, 30 % of Germans and 12 % of Austrians stated that they themselves or a member of their family had experienced an incident occurring during a medical care measurement.
- Only 26 % of EU citizens, 33 % of Germans but 57 % of Austrians stated that they or the person in question had reported this incident.
- Of all those who had surgery or a family member receiving a surgical treatment, 67 % of EU citizens, 81 % of Austrians and 90 % of

Germans said that they had signed a statement of consent before the implementation of the treatment process.

- Questioned who they would turn to in order to submit a claim for compensation for a damage resulting from a medical treatment, participants replied as follows (multiple answers possible):
  - Lawyer: EU 48 %, AT 65 %, D 75 %
  - Hospital management: EU 37 %, D 56 %, AT 28 %
  - Institution for patient safety: EU 29 %, D 50 %, AT30 %
  - Consumer Protection Organization: EU 21 %, D 34 %, AT 27 %
  - Physician, health-care professional or pharmacist: EU 12 %, D 19 %, 10 %
- 70 % of EU citizens, 86 % of Germans and 95 % of Austrians rated the general quality of health care in their respective countries as good.

2.2.2   Selected Initiatives of German Medical Chambers for Implementation of "Patient Safety"

The "Zentralstelle der deutschen Ärzteschaft zur Qualitätssicherung in der Medizin" (Central Office of German Medical Profession for Quality Assurance in Medicine) was founded in 1995 and renamed the "Ärztliches Zentrum für Qualität in der Medizin" – ÄZQ (Agency for Quality Assurance in Medicine) – in 2003. The 108th German Medical Assembly passed extensive trailblazing decisions proposed under the agenda point VII "Medical error management/Patient safety". These included decisions on fundamental principles of development of patient safety from a physician's vantage, on the German Coalition for Patient Safety and the supplementation of the training curriculum in medical quality management, a constantly evolving national curriculum in its 4th edition (Bundesärztekammer 2007). The Hessen State Medical Chamber and most other regional

chambers have introduced additional education guidelines for physicians and offer respective training. The KBV, BÄK and ÄZQ (National Association of Statutory Health Insurance Physicians, the German Medical Association and the Agency for Quality Assurance in Medicine) have been promoting error reporting and learning systems since 2005/2006.

In 2009, the Council of the European Union issued "Recommendations on Patient Safety" divided into the following areas of emphasis:

1. Support of introduction and development of effective and comprehensive patient safety strategies
2. Patient empowerment and access to comprehensible information
3. Support of introduction and expansion of blame-free reporting and learning systems
4. Support of further of education and advanced training programmes for health-care workers on patient safety at their respective level (see Bundesärztekammer 2009)

2.2.3   The German Coalition for Patient Safety

The Aktionsbündnis Patientensicherheit e.V. (German Coalition for Patient Safety) was founded in Düsseldorf in 2005 with the support of various medical associations. It unites health-care professionals of various areas in the research, development and dissemination of methods aimed at improving patient safety and establishing effective risk management strategies in the health-care sector. It offers information and documentation such as recommendations for action or checklists to increase safety for surgical procedures, in print and online, for professionals as well as patients (www.aktionsbuendnis-patientensicherheit.de). The coalition participates in various national and international projects, including the "Aktion Saubere Hände" (Clean Hands Campaign), and issues an annual "Agenda Patient Safety" detailing their activities (www.patientensicherheit-online.de).

2.2.4 Important Terms and Definitions

Medical quality management views risk management as an integral part of its setup. Patient safety can generally be defined as the avoidance of adverse events in health care (Hoffmann and Rohe 2010). Such events can be divided into unpreventable and preventable events. Injuries stemming from preventable treatment mistakes are deemed as iatrogenic damages. Risk management further differentiates between active (such as intraoperative severing of a structure exempt of surgical plans) and latent (due to organizational deficiencies) human failures. The Swiss Cheese Model identifies error chains caused by spatial and temporal occurrences and illustrates the interaction of active and latent human failure.

The Coalition for Patient Safety in its statutes (Aktionsbündnis Patientensicherheit e.V. 2009) defines patient safety as follows: Patient safety is understood as the absence of adverse events and damages in health care, and the term risk management covers a range of methods aimed at minimizing undesired events and damages in health care.

2.2.5 Risk Management in Hospitals

The first systematic studies on the frequency of adverse incidents occurring in hospitals were conducted in the early 1990s (Brennan et al. 1991; Leape et al. 1991) in the USA. Results showed that 3.7 % of patients suffered from adverse incidents. Fifty-eight percent of these incidents were deemed, in principle, preventable. Checklists (such as the "Surgical Safety Checklist" recommended by the WHO in 2009) formulated to increase patient safety during surgical treatments were widely discussed, and their efficiency in error prevention was scientifically examined (Busemann et al. 2012; Fudickar et al. 2012).

A survey in German general acute hospitals with more than 50 beds by Blum et al. (2008) found that 19.9 % of hospitals reported that they were actively operating a clinical risk management system. Of the active process elements conducted, the most often mentioned ones were risk analysis and risk control. 84 % of hospitals with risk management were of the opinion that their measurements had improved patient safety.

In 2007/2008 and again 2010, a Swiss group of investigators from universities of Zürich and Luzern conducted two studies (standardized questionnaire, total responder rate 43 %. It is not unlikely that hospitals with already established in-house risk management systems might be overrepresented) dealing with clinical risk management (CRM) in 324/321 hospitals all over Switzerland (Briner et al. 2009; Briner 2011; Manser et al. 2007). By 2007/2008, clinical risk management (CRM) had been widely integrated into general quality management. 35 % of hospitals had committed to binding strategic goals specifically defined for CRM; an additional 28 % were planning to shortly implement such requirements. The so-called Second National Monitoring of Clinical Risk Management in 2010 described the important changes found, compared to 2007/2008:

- Increased number of hospitals with a centralized CRM coordination from 16 to 65 %.
- More hospitals (41 % compared to 34 %) had committed to clearly defined strategic specific goals for the execution of CRM. Tasks, competences and responsibilities in CRM had increasingly been defined and implemented, in a structured or unstructured format (64 % compared to 51 % in 2008).
- CRM teams were mostly made up by nurses (59 %) and physicians (54 %). Seventy percent of all professionals handling CRM measurements had completed quality management training.
- In 2010, 71 % of all participating Swiss hospitals utilized institution-wide reporting systems for critical incidents (incident reporting systems, IRS) and only 6 % had not implemented the system in any of their clinics. This implies that the usage of IRS by 2010 had been accepted as national common practice in Switzerland.
- Results regarding the optimization potential of CRM were similar to those of 2007/2008. These included training in patient safety and

standardization of methods and processes, clear definition of tasks, competences and responsibilities, open and honest handling of errors and weaknesses and maintaining regular exchange of information between central CRM and their associated clinics.

Lauterberg et al. (2012) reported a second study on 1815 German hospitals (responder rate 26.7 %) with more than 50 beds about the status of their clinical risk management in 2010. Some interesting findings were:

- Hospitals rarely employed expert personnel exclusively responsible for CRM.
- Only 15 % of hospitals had personnel tasked with CRM responsibility in all departments/clinics/functional areas.
- 48 % of hospitals had access to a local CIRS (Critical Incident Reporting System) with 35.5 % actively using the system. Reporting incidents anonymously was almost uniformly possible.
- Systematic collation of the results of risk analysis for various areas such as infection protection, medication safety or surgical complications was conducted by less than half of the hospitals surveyed.
- Surveyed clinics reported a need for extensive CRM training for their personnel.

2.2.6   Improving Patient Rights (Patient Rights Law) in 2013

2013 saw by law the implementation (Patientenrechtegesetz 2013) of reporting requirements concerning risk management and incident reporting systems as part of quality reporting in hospitals. Furthermore, the new law reveals one of the main problems physicians have had to deal with unsuccessfully: how to effectively convey important information to individual patients so they have fully understood their respective situations and how to monitor and document the understanding of such communication. Already before the new legislation, physicians were complaining

about the continuously evolving stricter bureaucratic and formal requirements for patient information and such documentation.

Experience of state chambers of physicians with patient complaints has shown that many of those patients who feel mistreated or are discontent with their diagnosis or therapy, or feel personally insulted by how they were treated by their physician, often directly approach this physician before they consult a lawyer, association, consumer organization or institution. Many physicians, however, experience difficulties accepting the charges against them and so miss the chance to start an open and cooperative communication process instead of rejecting any accusatory remarks (Aktionsbündnis Patientensicherheit e.V. 2011). Physicians also often mistakenly assume that they will lose the support of their professional liability insurers when admitting any type of error. Physician's reluctance or denial to share or hand over patient files often leads to additional aggression and conflict readiness on the patient's side and can be avoided.

References

Aktionsbündnis Patientensicherheit e.V. (2009) Satzung i.d.F.v. 4. Juli 2009. www.aktionsbuendnis-patientensicherheit.de

Aktionsbündnis Patientensicherheit e.V. (2011) Reden ist Gold – Kommunikation nach einem Zwischenfall. Bonn. www.aktionsbuendnis-patientensicherheit.de

Blum K et al (2008) Krankenhaus Barometer Umfrage 2008. Deutsches Krankenhausinstitut e.V, Düsseldorf

Brennan TA et al (1991) Incidence of adverse events and negligence in hospitalized patients: results of the Harvard Medical Practice Study I. N Eng J Med 324:370–376

Briner M (2011) Zweites nationales Monitoring zum klinischen Risikomanagement im Spital. Zusammenfassung der Ergebnisse. Schweizerische Ärztezeitung 92(12):463–466

Briner M et al (2009) Erste Schweizer Erhebung zum klinischen Risikomanagement im Spital. Schweizerische Ärztezeitung 90(15/16):635–638

Bundesärztekammer (2007) Curriculum Ärztliches Qualitätsmanagement 4. Auflage www.bundesaerztekammer.de

Bundesärztekammer (2009) Empfehlungen des Rates der Europäischen Union zur Sicherheit der Patienten vom 5. Juni 2009 – Umsetzung von Patientensicherheit in Deutschland. www.bundesaerztekammer.de

Bundesärztekammer (2015a) Gutachterkommissionen und Schlichtungsstellen bei den Ärztekammern. www. undesaerztekammer.de

Bundesärztekammer (2015b) Statistische Erhebung der Gutachterkommissionen und Schlichtungsstellen für das Statistikjahr 2013. www.bundesaerztekammer.de

Busemann A et al (2012) Einführung von Operations-checklisten als Teil des Risikomanagements. Chirurg 83(7):611–616

Deutscher Ärztetag (2005) Entschließungen zum Tagesordnungspunkt VII Beschlußprotokoll des 108. Deutschen Ärztetages. Deutsches Ärzteblatt 102(19) A: 1379–1381. Auch verfügbar unter: www.bundesaerztekammer.de

Fudickar A et al (2012) „Surgical Safety Checklist"der Weltgesundheitsorganisation. Deutsches Ärzteblatt 109(42):695–701

Gesetz zur Verbesserung der Rechte von Patientinnen und Patienten (Patientenrechtegesetz) 2013 BR-Drs: 007–13. www.bmg.bund.de

Hoffmann B, Rohe J (2010) Patientensicherheit und Fehlermanagement. Deutsches Ärzteblatt 107(6): 92–99

Kohn LT, Corrigan JM, Donaldson MS (eds) (2000) To err is human. Building a safer health system. National Academy Press, Washington, DC

Landesärztekammer (2015) Wegweiser für das Verfahren vor der Gutachter- und Schlichtungsstelle der Landesärztekammer Hessen. www.laekh.de

Lauterberg J et al (2012) Befragung zum Einführungsstand von klinischem Risikomanagement (kRM) in deutschen Krankenhäusern (Abschlußbericht). Institut für Patientensicherheit Bonn also in: www. aktionsbuendnis-patientensicherheit.de

Leape LL et al (1991) The nature of adverse events in hospitalized patients. Results of the Harvard Medical Practice Study II. N Eng J Med 324:377–384

Manser T et al (2007) Klinisches Risikomanagement in Schweizer Spitälern. Schweizerische Ärztezeitung 88(51/52):2168–2169

Scheppokat K-D (2009) Verlässlichkeit der Bewertungen ist unzureichend. Deutsches Ärzteblatt 106(20): A980–A984

Scheppokat KD, Neu J (2007) Medizinische Daten und Qualitätsmanagement. Deutsches Ärzteblatt 104(46): A3172–A3177

TNS Opinion & Social (2010) Patientensicherheit und Qualität der medizinischen Versorgung. Spezial Eurobarometer 327/Welle 72.2 Brüssel. http://ec. europa.eu/public_opinion/index_en.htm

Human Behavior in the Execution of Tasks: Influencing Factors of Decision-Making

Dirk-Matthias Rose

Abstract

Making mistakes is part of general human behavior. This chapter gives an insight into the processes of the human brain and explains why and how we think and behave. Specific forms of human behavior are the reasons why specific methods of process management have developed.

3.1 Introduction

All people have to continually make decisions. These decisions may be wrong or right; as a consequence, they may generate or prevent damage. Therefore, the knowledge of how an individual makes decisions and how decision-making can be influenced is an important factor in the risk management of an enterprise, particularly in the public health sector.

Frequently in the public health sector, decision-making has to be done quickly without an adequate basis for decision-making. A life-threatening situation, however, requires prompt decisions regarding life-saving treatments without information about the medical history or without laboratory values.

As a car driver, you always make decisions without intentional decision-making, but with automaticity in the appropriate situation (e.g., declutching). Automated decisions are the result of the intensive exercising of behavioral patterns. They are executed in the subcortical areas of the brain and the main advantage is their velocity. Unexpected situations require a cortical analysis to evoke a proper reaction. These reactions are the results of analytical processes in the brain. They need a significantly longer execution time than automated reactions. If the brain can rely on empirical values, a knowledge-based decision is possible. In the absence of empirical values, an intuitive decision, which relies on general (life) experience and emotions, is necessary. If many critical decisions have to be made simultaneously or sequentially, an overload of the brain's capacity could occur. Mistakes or absurd displacement activities would be the result.

D.-M. Rose, MD, PhD
Institut für Lehrergesundheit am Institut für,
Arbeits-, Sozial- und Umweltmedizin,
Universitätsmedizin der Johannes-Gutenberg-
Universität Mainz, Kupferbergterrasse 17-19,
Mainz 55116, Germany
e-mail: dirk-matthias.rose@universitaetsmedizin-mainz.de

© Springer-Verlag Berlin Heidelberg 2016
W. Merkle (ed.), *Risk Management in Medicine*, DOI 10.1007/978-3-662-47407-5_3

An example of this can be found in the history of two aircraft accidents. In the first case, shortly after takeoff, the flameout of both engines was due to bird strikes. Normally in this situation, the aircraft crashes and causes the loss of the lives of many passengers. However, the pilot and his co-pilot were able to successfully ditch on the Hudson River without the loss of a single life. As the pilot pointed out in his book, the decision to perform an action that had never been performed before (ditching on the Hudson River) relied on his excellent knowledge of the aircraft's technology, the clear assignment of responsibilities and duties within the team, the pilot ignoring and blocking his own emotions (fear for his life), and naturally the good luck that there were favorable circumstances (Sullenberger and Zaslow 2009).

In the second case, an aircraft crashed over the Atlantic Ocean. Emotional decisions (fear of the financial consequences of an extra landing required to avoid a zone of bad weather) prompted actions that led to technical problems, including failure of many instruments owing to weather problems (i.e., icing). Normally, an accident could have been avoided by following basic flying rules (maintaining the proper pitch of the aircraft without current information about altitude and speed to avoid stalling, which is what finally happened; see Chap. 5). However, extreme strain and stress, the flight crew's inexperience with this type of aircraft, and the inconclusive assignment of responsibilities, resulted in unreproducible spurious actions, ignored warnings, and an inconsistent series of decisions. In total, these mistakes caused the aircraft to crash and kill all of the passengers.

Therefore, it is important to have knowledge of the factors influencing decision-making in humans and the resulting actions, to control these factors so as to optimize reactions and decision-making under the auspices of minimizing risk. Despite an enormous gain in knowledge in the recent past, it is not yet clear in which regions of the brain decision-making is located or how decision-making functions. It is not clear why one human is decisive or tends to avoid decision-making. Functional neuroimaging with MRT shows individual differences in decision-making, comparing normal employees with managers, who have jobs involving making decisions faster and more frequently (Caspers et al. 2012).

In this chapter, the different influencing factors on human decision-making, the resulting actions, and the chance to change these pathways are presented.

3.2 Factors Influencing Decision-Making

Decision-making is influenced by external and individual factors. Basically, a decision is made by weighing up benefit and damage, advantage and disadvantage, and effort and gain. All these factors are influenced by terms and conditions, one's own capabilities and emotional estimations, and ratings based on one's own life experience. These factors are highlighted in more detail.

3.2.1 Organizational Preconditions (Hard and Soft Facts)

Organizational preconditions summarize different hard and soft facts. Hard facts mean all factors that are structural and infrastructural specified (see the section "Hard Facts"). Soft facts mean the functioning of the organization, in particular its philosophy and organizational structure (see the section "Soft Facts").

3.2.1.1 Hard Facts

Based on the example of a hospital, the hard facts are the infrastructure, the technical and staff resources responsible for the operational availability of materials and personnel.

Hard facts are also the professional qualifications of the personnel, the binding rules of continuing education, the implementation of knowledge-based guidelines, and the transfer of internal quality management requirements.

As a consequence, time factors and specified levels of treatment performance, care, and follow-up of patients are generated.

Hard facts are determined, documented, and revisable. Deviations of specifications should be determined by risk management. The control of nonconformity is established by the nomination of a person in charge to determine time frames within which deviations are to be eliminated. With periodic review, hard facts should be adapted to changes in workflows or to new requirements.

Technical and personal resources are the basic requirements for adequate decisions and actions. Even a highly qualified and motivated cardiac surgeon cannot perform cardiac surgery without an adequately equipped operating theater and qualified staff.

3.2.1.2 Soft Facts

Soft facts are substantially affected by corporate philosophy. This includes organizations with flat or distinct control hierarchies, an obligatory and transparent planning process, operating schedules, and standards. Even the continuity of management and the necessary settlement of subsequent operations are included in the soft facts that influence the decision-making and activities of the personnel.

Communication in an organization is also critical. Adequate, customized, and comprehensive information is an integral part of a positive corporate culture that motivates performance and staff activities positively. Rumors and watchwords are frequently obstructive to performance.

In areas in which critical or risk-related decisions have to be made, fault management is very important, as the main aim is to learn from mistakes, near faults or near accidents, and not to sanction them (see Chaps. 1, 8, and 9).

Fault management covers various fields:

1. Fault could be avoided by routine skill-based exercises. The procedures are depicted by standard operating procedures (SOPs) or flowcharts. New personnel undergo training continuously during their period of vocational adjustment. For example, new surgical techniques are practiced on phantoms or the handling of critical flight behavior is taught in a flight simulator (see Chap. 6).
2. Faults could be minimized if a mistake is ascertained and a solution is found. If the same or a related problem recurs, it will be solved quickly (rule-based). Typically, checklists comply with these requirements, to work off an intermittent failure during a flight in civil aviation, or the counting of instruments, needles, and swabs before and after surgical intervention (see Chap. 6).
3. Complex faults resulting from the interactions of many factors with different specifications could be handled by knowledge-based solutions. An example of a knowledge-based solution is the corporate case conference. However, knowledge databases, or "if–then" decision rules, could contribute systematically to minimizing failures (see Chaps. 11 and 13).

Internal and external factors of the corporate environment are soft facts. Also, the health management of a company relies partly on soft facts in maintaining the performance of the personnel.

Furthermore, operational, political, social, and familial environments may positively or negatively support commitment, reliability, and endorsement.

Beneath the individual factors, environmental factors may strengthen individual calmness, and feelings of security, optimism, and confidence. Disruptive factors and negative impacts in this area, combined with time pressure and pressure to perform, especially in a hospital environment, may not only provoke negative effects on the performance of the medical staff, but may also have a crabwise effect on patient satisfaction.

3.2.2   Personal Requirements (Hard and Soft Skills)

Beneath the external setting, individual capabilities and expertise play an important role. Personal skills are partly hereditary, but can often be learned, amended, and checked. The individual's personality plays a substantial role, can only partly be influenced and interferes with emotions, of which we are only partially aware. Frequently, it is not be possible to have complete control over these factors. However, briefing could be achieved to inform about the hazards of involuntary misinterpretation and knee-jerk reactions. Consequently, it is possible to recognize these hazards and to potentially avoid them.

3.2.2.1 Hard Skills

Hard skills regarding our decisions and actions are beneath other skills: intelligence, analytical thinking, professional expertise, specific skills from education, advanced training, professional experience, and the capability for risk analysis and fault analysis. Most of these factors can be learned or improved by training and can be measured and tested. The test results could be used for the specific assignment or the definition of required further education.

3.2.2.2 Soft Skills

Particularly in a team, beneath the professional qualifications, the so called "soft skills" are also absolutely necessary for success (see Chap. 14). The ability to communicate, the capacity for teamwork, and the ability to manage conflict are necessary in a team, especially for managing a team. You need fluency, but also emotional intelligence and cross-cultural competence. To manage a team, knowledge of human nature, give-and-take, empathy, and to setting a good example are necessary soft skills. These skills could stimulate the whole team to perform at its best. Without these skills, the performance of the team could be negatively impaired by, for example, mobbing or distrust, and could lead to uncertainty, concern, anxiety, stress, agitation, and consequently irredeemable.

Individual training can be provided for many of these factors. Time, stress, and conflict management can be learned to a certain extent. Particular individual coaching of managers (see Chap. 7) is helpful to improve these skills, which are essential for successful management.

The management board of a hospital carries out a substantial part of a functional risk management by establishing positive or less positive general conditions for "team hospital" (see Chap. 1).

However, these factors are influenced in the current situation by individual emotions, which are involuntary and can only be controlled in a limited way.

3.2.3 Emotions

Emotions are affected by life experiences and develop differently in individuals. Izard (2009) and Izard et al. (2008) differentiate among ten basic emotions. Only happiness and interest are rated as positive; the other emotions, namely, fright, disregard, shame, guilt, fear, disgust, grief, and anger, are rated as negative.

Emotions influence our decisions and operations significantly. They occur automatically and rapidly and are a part of our evolved strategy for survival. Nowadays, they are frequently counterproductive, however, and seduce us into positions and operations that are not adequate for the prevailing situation. As they cannot be controlled directly, one can try to prevent the effects of emotions with suitable training. This is very effective, particularly if the causes can be influenced by therapy (e.g., arachnophobia or fear of flying). Often, it is only possible to explain how emotions influence our cognition, inducing us to make wrong decisions or act in an inadequate manner.

Emotions, and their influence on our behavior, attitudes, decisions, and operations, are the subject of current psychological research. Brain research locates, with the use of functional brain mapping (MRT, SPECT), the area of the brain in which observed activities can be matched to specific emotions.

Emotions develop early in life. Newborns do not have self-awareness and social behavior, but these develop between the 18th and 24th month of life. At the age of 4 years the child is able to pick up on the emotional constitution of other people without any emotional indicators such as crying or screaming. This is called mentalizing or perspective-taking, and is part of the "theory of mind" (ToM) (Blair 2005) and cognitive empathy. A substantial part of emotional and affective empathy takes place in the mirror neurons. They are essential for the emotional dyeing of the mimics and the kinesthetic expression received from the vis-à-vis (Blair 2005). Dysfunction of the mirror neurons system and the processing of the signals in the amygdala seem to be connected to autism (e.g., the absence of empathy) (Britton et al. 2006).

Emotions substantially influence the cognition affected by one's own subjective or irrational comprehension and thereby risk analyses. Thus, individuals rate risks in very different ways (see Chap. 6). The risk perception of an expert differs significantly from that of an ordinary person and could cause different actions. Therefore, either the overestimation of one's own capabilities or technical options (overconfidence; see Chap. 4), or a reserved and observant attitude, leading to a situation that is critical or no longer controllable over time, could generate fatal consequences.

Strong emotions in critical situations require a high degree of self-control. Self-control, however, depends on the brain's available energy resources. Strong emotional stress reduces the blood glucose level. A low level of blood glucose after a tough activity, such as self-control, leads to successively decreasing performance. A dose of glucose rapidly increases performance (Gailliot et al. 2007). Consumption of glucose during tough emotional self-control (thoughts of suicide) could lead to a "protective" self-regulating fatigue (Gailliot et al. 2006), which is not desirable in successful crisis management.

3.3 Where Do Decisions Arise? New Aspects of Brain Research

With improvement in the time-based resolution of imaging techniques it is now possible to watch action-activated brain areas simultaneously with functional magnetic resonance imaging (fMRI). Thus, an imaging technique may be more precise than EEG in illustrating activated brain areas. This technique is amended by the possibility of the determination of a neurotransmitter, such as serotonin, glutathione, and noradrenaline. Other techniques, such as positron emission tomography (PET), single –photon emission computed tomography (SPECT) or cranial computed tomography (cCT), can detect damaged regions of the brain, but are too slow in their time-based resolution to detect process flows or decision-making in the brains of healthy people. These techniques are also problematic because of radiation exposure.

Current publications provide increasing evidence for which functions are located in different significant brain regions. Table 3.1 sums up some of these results.

3.3.1 Functional Magnetic Resonance Imaging

Functional magnetic resonance imaging (fMRI) has been used in recent years and a couple of studies have been published that monitored different brain areas to find out where ethical decision-making and social cognition happen. One aspect of this topic is the ToM, defined as "the competency to make an assumption of activities of awareness in another person and recognize these activities in the own person" (Fonagy and Bateman 2006). This theory, amongst others, is important for the development of social skills and the ability to empathize.

Normally, fMRI uses the possibility of differentiating blood with high oxygen content from blood with low oxygen content (BOLD imaging) and thus differentiating activated from non-activated brain regions.

3.3.2 Transmitter as Messenger Substances

Among the locations of brain areas involved in the genesis and processing of decisions, operations, and emotions, neural transmitters play an important role in the characteristics or categorical orientation of decisions and emotional rating that is nowadays not fully understood. Dopamine-, serotonin-, and glutamate-dependent receptors are influenced in an oppositional manner, whereby different individual genetic specificities could lead to completely different decisions, while the given situation and the activated areas of the brain are identical.

Dopamine is a widespread neurotransmitter in the central nervous system. Two classes of dopamine-dependent receptors could arbitrate either excitatory or inhibitory signals. Dopamine is crucial to target-oriented behavior, cognition,

Table 3.1 Assignment of activities in brain regions to functions and emotions

Abbreviation of brain region	Designation of the brain region	Activation-influenced functions/emotions/ transmitter	Reference
ACC	Anterior cingulate cortex	At the dorsal part: weighing up between the relative worthiness of an acute decision and the greatest worthiness in the long-term view, a high level of activity in the case of decisions with a high degree of uncertainty, in connection with alertness and self-confidence, emotional recognition of facial expression (sadness) Emotionally hypo-reactive (criminal) individuals show significantly more risky behavior and anticipation of punishment compared with normal individuals	(Boorman et al. 2013; Britton et al. 2006; Causse et al. 2013; Prehn et al. 2013)
A	Amygdala	Activation in the case of anxiety, disgust (in particular, olfactory, fear, sadness [recognition of emotions from facial expressions]) Serotonin intensifies the activation in the case of a negative experience, to process this negative experience in future productive behavior and risk-avoidance	(Britton et al. 2006; Gottfried et al. 2002, 2003; Wicker et al. 2003; Macoveanu et al. 2012)
aTC	Anterior temporal cortex	Emotional activation during annoyance (suspected to be dopamine-dependent)	
DLPFC	Dorsolateral prefrontal cortex	High level of activity at a high degree of uncertainty; in floundering individuals a lower level of activity with more risky behavior in the same situation	(Causse et al. 2013)
INS	Insula	Activation of mirror neurons assessing incoming information emotionally, arousal by disgust and disgusting odors and flavors, significantly reduced activation in obese individuals (BMI > 30)	(Rizzolatti et al. 2008; Wicker et al. 2003; Hendrick et al. 2012)
IPL	Inferior parietal lobe	Social estimation, empathy-based estimation of the gap between one's own and third-party interests	(Janowski et al. 2013)
MPFC	Medial prefrontal cortex	Empathic options, triggered by the IPL, integrated into the process of the appreciation of the intentions of others, empathic assessment of the gestures of others (mimic, finger gestures); serotonin reduces the reaction to negative incidents	(Janowski et al. 2013; Lindenberg et al. 2012; Macoveanu et al. 2012)
STS	Superior temporal sulcus	Triggering of emotions by gestures (movements of hands)	(Lindenberg et al. 2012)
VMPFC	Ventromedial prefrontal cortex	Decision between the chosen and the next best option at every intermediate step of decision-making, important link region in complex motoric decision processes to the medial motor cortex	(Boorman et al. 2013; Madlon-Kay et al. 2013)
PMC	Premotoric cortex	Mirror neurons triggered activation by anger (recognition of emotions at facial expression)	(Pichon et al. 2009; Grèzes et al. 2007; van Heijnsbergen et al. 2007; Adolphs 2002a, b)

concentration, and a reward attitude (Klein 2011). Genetic variations of dopamine ToM genes (Blair 2005) lead to different forms of approval-seeking behavior and could pre-dispose to neuropsychiatric abnormalities (Dreher 2013). Unforeseen aversive events and rewards lead to a significant signal of prediction bias by dopaminergic neurons with activation of a network in the striatum, the front insula, and the anterior cingulate cortex (ACC) (Metereau and Dreher 2013), which induces a learning effect boosted by reward and punishment.

Glutamate is the most important excitatory neurotransmitter and is found in different densities in all brain structures (Klein 2011). There is little understanding of its function. It seems that it plays an important role in attention- and memory-relevant processes and is essential for learning.

Risk-avoiding behavior is triggered by serotonin-dependent receptors. The inhibition of the re-uptake of serotonin (increasing the blood concentration of serotonin) leads to stronger reactions of the negative outcomes of risky behavior (Grady et al. 2013; Macoveanu et al. 2012). Also, fear, aggression, and suicidality are influenced by the neural transmitter serotonin (Fisher and Hariri 2013; Bortolato et al. 2013; Crockett et al. 2010).

The interdependencies of the different neural transmitter systems are largely ambiguous, whereas polymorphism and genetic variations cause various individual reactions.

3.4 Influence of Facts, Skills, and Emotions on Subjective Risk Sensitivity and Decision-Making

Beneath the biological basis for the factors are involved why and when different decisions will be made. Individual education and experience and the external variables and incidents that have been experienced by having emotions are the basis of individual decision profiles.

Decisions have been very important for survival throughout evolution. Many decisions have to be made quickly to avoid harassment, damage or death. These decisions are triggered by emotions, experiences, and instincts, and are executed automatically and not controlled by willful decision-making. Their advantage is their velocity and decision-making with the risk to be at fault in this situation owing to misjudgment.

Up to now, ethical decision-making has led to the open question of whether this decision-making due to:

- Rational considerations, or
- Emotional and intuitive effects, or
- Progresses successively with education and experience from relational consideration to intuitive action.

Certainly during infantile development, ethics and moral beliefs are adopted from adult attachment figures (psychological parents; authority-branded infantile realism). With growing development these beliefs become independent from psychological parents and further develop to become self-determined, autonomous ethics (Piaget 1990). Even social interactions are branded ethical decisions. According to the Haidt's model, emotions and affective intuition are held accountable for actions, but they are first "post-hoc" after the decision made has been defended with willful considerations and cognitive skills (Hauser 2006, 2007).

Greene et al. (2001, 2004) and Greene and Haidt (2002) developed for complex ethical dilemma decisions (meaning decisions that lead to an undesired result) the conflict–control model, where emotions highlight decision options with a feeling of acceptance or denial. If emotions and decision options are congruent, the reaction time is not prolonged by reflections or considerations. If emotions and decision options are not congruent, the reaction time is prolonged, as higher cognitive brain areas are activated to evaluate the decision options again.

3.4.1 Influence of Facts on Decisions

External circumstances (facilities, work conditions, and work organization) are basic requirements for providing proper and adequate work.

3.4.2 Influence of Skills on Decisions

One's own skills and the knowledge of these skills increase self-confidence and the willingness to decide. Test participants with a greater working memory have been more self-confident and less influenced by negative feedback compared with pro-bands with a smaller working memory (Schmeichel and Demaree 2010). Greater intellectual power cor-relates with less of an emotional reaction to adequate emotional stimuli (Schmeichel et al. 2008). Therefore, a good education with a high level of (job-related) experience is the best protection against emotional burdens, with a risk of non-adequate reactions and of exhaustion and delayed decision-making.

3.4.3 Influence of Emotions on Decisions

Many decisions are made quickly and automati-cally. They are reactions to external impressions that prompt action, and are based on emotions and predefine options of acting. The greatest ambition is to avoid deprivation and ensure sur-vival (anxiety-based decisions). Therefore, per-manent misjudgments occur owing to errors of reasoning and cognition. These errors lead to spurious actions, if advantages and disadvantages of an action are not calculated promptly. Some well-known faults are listed in Table 3.2. These are only a few examples of misjudgments sys-tematically caused by emotions (Dobelli 2011).

3.5 How Can the Process of Decision-Making Be Improved and Where Are the Limits? The Influence of Human Behavior as Part of Risk Management

Emotions are responsible either for quick deci-sions or for completely wrong interpretations of the prevailing situation. Thus, a tendency exists toward decision-making based on one's own experiences that have been gained under a strong

Table 3.2 Systematic false conclusions and their sources

Type of error	Source
Fear of deprivation	To avoid deprivations/losses one takes snowballing hazards, if there is a minimal chance of avoiding deprivation (keeping stock)
Impact bias	Overestimation of one's own feelings
Anecdotal fallacy	Cognitive misjudgment, as one believes more strongly in field reports than in statistical evidence. This applies particularly to one's own experience with strong emotional impressions
Post-hoc fallacy	To manage the daily flood of information, partial information is complemented autonomously without a survey of all the possible solutions
Situational bias	Varying assessment of risks depending on the ambience
Confirmation bias	One-sided selection or interpretation of information to confirm one's own rating (failure blindness)
Authority bias	Trusting authorities, even it is rational or ethically absurd. Effective counter-measure is, e.g., crew resource management
Overconfidence effect	Systematic overestimation of one's own skills and of one's own knowledge; more distinct in men than in women
Survivorship bias	Systematic overestimation of the chance of success, as failures do not become as public as successes

emotional influence by ignoring logical facts. Because decisions and actions, especially in the medical sector, are made or initialized under strong emotional burdens, mishandling and fail-ure are more probable in this area than in others.

3.5.1 Creating a Setting of Failure Prevention: Workplace Ergonomy

The reliability of finding equipment and tools in the usual places improves and accelerates workflows. Thus, errors can be avoided. For experts in particular, an unergonomic workplace and bad workflow organization could cause errors. A study showed that the recognition of references in an experienced individual occurred more quickly than in the inexperienced, if these references appeared in the assumed places. If these references did not appear in the assumed places, however, recognition by experts was worse than that in non-experts (Borowsky et al. 2008). Reliable workplace surroundings with predictable workflows contribute significantly to the minimization of failure.

3.5.2 Learning and Practice: Error Management Training

Scientific studies constrain what has been best practice for millennia. Automated processes proceed quickly and without time-consuming reflection. Managers, used to frequent decision-making, look for rule-based proceedings and therefore to the automation of decision-making. These processes are transferred in subcortical regions of the brain and occur faster than in non-managers (Caspers et al. 2012). However, this procedure risks using false rules, consequently leading to the wrong decisions. This risk could be improved by the chance to learn from errors (error management training). The chance to make errors without anxiety leads to the improvement of processing and the comprehension of information. Thus, learning from errors could accelerate knowledge uptake (see Chap. 8).

3.5.3 Rule-Based Performance

Particularly in critical situations, quick and correct decisions are necessary. As specified, decision-making is highly negatively influenced by anxiety, disgust, anger, and other emotions, and even disrupts actions in extreme situations. Also, trained skills could be totally blocked. In this situation it is extremely helpful to rely on role-based actions and workflows. This provides some degree of certainty in decision-making.

In commercial aviation, for example, completion of checklists is standard procedure in critical situations (e.g., flameout of an engine) and enhances flight safety.

Rule-based performance results in quicker decisions and is can be learned and taught. Thus, compared with non-experts, experts are able to make faster and more energy-efficient decisions (Caspers et al. 2012). The implementation of SOPs in hospitals should support these efforts.

3.5.4 Communication and Team-Oriented Decision-Making

In hospitals a team (consisting of nurses and doctors) is usually involved in the treatment of a patient. The cooperation of all the staff involved could significantly improve a patient's health. In reality, the situation is frequently different (Bharwani et al. 2012). A study of four different teams (three of which had been organized hierarchically) in a typical academic hospital showed that there was no team work. The ward physicians communicated only with the senior physician. The nurses and other nonmedical personnel did not make any proposals, did not communicate, and assumed that their work would be coordinated with the work and decisions of the physicians by others (see Chap. 14). This approach differs significantly from that of successful teams (Bharwani et al. 2012).

To create successful teams in the medical sector, the preconditions have to be improved. Therefore, teams need time for team meetings to discuss their proposals together. Structured protocols of team meetings promote the participation of all team members. The meetings should take place in a calm and stress-free environment. The members of the team need to be trained in team-work and coached periodically (see Chap. 7). In commercial aviation, crew members are frequently trained in collaboration and communication skills (crew coordination; see Chap. 14), and this training has improved accident prevention. The longer the teams stayed together, the better their team success has been, if the rules implemented have been respected.

Conclusion

The concurrence of many factors leads to decisions and initiated actions. Not all contributing factors can be taught, acquired, prepared, audited or controlled equally or completely. However, all the skills, taken together, reduce the risk of incorrect decisions or critical actions.

Technical or organizational hard facts can be predetermined, planned, and verified. This means that in a hospital or doctor's office, the technical and structural requirements, the equipment, and periodic survey and servicing are carried out according to a structured schedule based on risk analysis. The organizational workflows (soft facts) can be planned, optimized, and taught because of experience gained from critical situations. Ergonomic procedures have to be compiled, reviewed, optimized, and strictly adhered to, so as to become operative and to avoid faults.

The continuous practice and amendment of individual skills (hard and soft skills) raise self-confidence and self-efficacy. The better trained and more experienced an expert is, the better and more effective are his scopes of action in critical situations requiring diverse parallel decisions and actions. The successful training of automated operations and processes and the practice of rule-based decisions in critical situations and on unforeseen occasions contribute to a reduction of anxiety and to confidence in successful solutions. Therefore, an overload with the risk of freezing decisions will occur significantly later.

As systematic team training with team coordination for situations in which the team has to work together improves competence in solving critical situations. In the medical sector, this makes a significant contribution to the safety of patients and the prevention of faults.

Emotionally affected learning outcomes and individual personality remain only hardly to affect sources of errors, especially in critical situations. The teaching and improvement of skills, facts, communication, and teamwork should help managers to recognize possible sources of errors and previous spurious actions and to minimize them by taking appropriate counteractive measures (automatization, rule-based decision-making, communication, and team management).

References

Adolphs R (2002a) Neural systems for recognizing emotion. Curr Opin Neurobiol 12(2):169–177

Adolphs R (2002b) Recognizing emotion from facial expressions: psychological and neurological mechanisms. Behav Cogn Neurosci Rev 1(1):21–62

Bharwani AM, Harris GC, Southwick FS (2012) Perspective: a business school view of medical interprofessional rounds: transforming rounding groups into rounding teams. Acad Med 87(12):1768–1771

Blair RJR (2005) Responding to the emotions of others: dissociating forms of empathy through the study of typical and psychiatric populations. Conscious Cogn 14(4):698–718

Boorman ED, Rushworth MF, Behrens TE (2013) Ventromedial prefrontal and anterior cingulate cortex adopt choice and default reference frames during sequential multi-alternative choice. J Neurosci 33(6):2242–2253

Borowsky A, Shinar D, Parmet Y (2008) The relation between driving experience and recognition of road signs relative to their locations. Hum Factors 50(2):173–182

Bortolato M, Pivac N, Muck Seler D, Nikolac Perkovic M, Pessia M, Di Giovanni G (2013) The role of the serotonergic system at the interface of aggression and suicide. Neuroscience 236:160–185

Britton JC, Phan KL, Taylor SF, Welsh RC, Berridge KC, Liberzon I (2006) Neural correlates of social and non-social emotions: an fMRI study. Neuroimage 31(1):397–409

Caspers S, Heim S, Lucas MG, Stephan E, Fischer L, Amunts K, Zilles K (2012) Dissociated neural processing for decisions in managers and non-managers. PLoS ONE 7(8):e43537

Causse M, Péran P, Dehais F, Caravasso CF, Zeffiro T, Sabatini U, Pastor J (2013) Affective decision making under uncertainty during a plausible aviation task: an fMRI study. Neuroimage 71:19–29

Crockett MJ, Clark L, Hauser MD, Robbins TW (2010) Serotonin selectively influences moral judgment and behavior through effects on harm aversion. Proc Natl Acad Sci U S A 107(40):17433–17438

Dobelli R (2011) Die Kunst des klaren Denkens. 52 Denkfehler, die Sie besser anderen überlassen. Hanser, München

Dreher J-C (2013) Neural coding of computational factors affecting decision making. Prog Brain Res 202:289–320

Fisher PM, Hariri AR (2013) Identifying serotonergic mechanisms underlying the corticolimbic response to threat in humans. Philos Trans R Soc Lond B Biol Sci 368(1615):20120192

Fonagy P, Bateman AW (2006) Mechanisms of change in mentalization-based treatment of BPD. J Clin Psychol 62(4):411–430

Gailliot MT, Schmeichel BJ, Baumeister RF (2006) Self-regulatory processes defend against the threat of death: effects of self-control depletion and trait self-control on thoughts and fears of dying. J Pers Soc Psychol 91(1):49–62

Gailliot MT, Baumeister RF, DeWall CN, Maner JK, Plant EA, Tice DM et al (2007) Self-control relies on glucose as a limited energy source: willpower is more than a metaphor. J Pers Soc Psychol 92(2):325–336

Gottfried JA, O'Doherty J, Dolan RJ (2002) Appetitive and aversive olfactory learning in humans studied using event-related functional magnetic resonance imaging. J Neurosci 22(24):10829–10837

Gottfried JA, O'Doherty J, Dolan RJ (2003) Encoding predictive reward value in human amygdala and orbitofrontal cortex. Science 301(5636):1104–1107

Grady CL, Siebner HR, Hornboll B, Macoveanu J, Paulson OB, Knudsen GM (2013) Acute pharmacologically induced shifts in serotonin availability abolish emotion-selective responses to negative face emotions in distinct brain networks. Eur Neuropsychopharmacol 23(5):368–378

Greene J, Haidt J (2002) How (and where) does moral judgment work? Trends Cogn Sci (Regul Ed) 6(12): 517–523

Greene JD, Sommerville RB, Nystrom LE, Darley JM, Cohen JD (2001) An fMRI investigation of emotional engagement in moral judgment. Science 293(5537):2105–2108

Greene JD, Nystrom LE, Engell AD, Darley JM, Cohen JD (2004) The neural bases of cognitive conflict and control in moral judgment. Neuron 44(2):389–400

Grèzes J, Pichon S, de Gelder B (2007) Perceiving fear in dynamic body expressions. Neuroimage 35(2):959–967

Hauser MD (2006) The liver and the moral organ. Soc Cogn Affect Neurosci 1(3):214–220

Hauser M (2007) What's fair? The unconscious calculus of our moral faculty. Novartis Found Symp 278: 41–50; discussion 50–5, 89–96, 216–21

Hendrick OM, Luo X, Zhang S, Li C-SR (2012) Saliency processing and obesity: a preliminary imaging study of the stop signal task. Obesity (Silver Spring) 20(9):1796–1802

Izard CE (2009) Emotion theory and research: highlights, unanswered questions, and emerging issues. Annu Rev Psychol 60:1–25

Izard C, Stark K, Trentacosta C, Schultz D (2008) Beyond emotion regulation: emotion utilization and adaptive functioning. Child Dev Perspect 2(3):156–163

Janowski V, Camerer C, Rangel A (2013) Empathic choice involves vmPFC value signals that are modulated by social processing implemented in IPL. Soc Cogn Affect Neurosci 8(2):201–208

Klein N (2011) Interaktion der Neurotransmitter Glutamat und Dopamin in belohnungsassoziierten Hirnstrukturen bei gesunden Menschen. Berlin, Medizinische Fakultät Charité – Universitätsmedizin Berlin, Berlin. Online verfügbar unter. http://nbn-resolving.de/urn: nbn:de:kobv:188-fudissthesis000000024995-2

Lindenberg R, Uhlig M, Scherfeld D, Schlaug G, Seitz RJ (2012) Communication with emblematic gestures: shared and distinct neural correlates of expression and reception. Hum Brain Mapp 33(4):812–823

Macoveanu J, Rowe JB, Hornboll B, Elliott R, Paulson OB, Knudsen GM, Siebner HR (2012) Playing it safe but losing anyway-Serotonergic signaling of negative outcomes in dorsomedial prefrontal cortex in the context of risk-aversion. Eur Neuropsychopharmacol. www.worldcat.org/oclc/889801425, doi: 10.1016/j. euroneuro.2012.09.006; Elsevier BV 2012-10-07

Madlon-Kay S, Pesaran B, Daw ND (2013) Action selection in multi-effector decision making. Neuroimage 70:66–79

Metereau E, Dreher J-C (2013) Cerebral correlates of salient prediction error for different rewards and punishments. Cereb Cortex 23(2):477–487

Piaget J (1990) Das moralische Urteil beim Kinde. 2. Aufl. München: Klett-Cotta im Dt. Taschenbuch-Verl (Dtv, 15015)

Pichon S, de Gelder B, Grèzes J (2009) Two different faces of threat. Comparing the neural systems for recognizing fear and anger in dynamic body expressions. Neuroimage 47(4):1873–1883

Prehn K, Schlagenhauf F, Schulze L, Berger C, Vohs K, Fleischer M et al (2013) Neural correlates of risk taking in violent criminal offenders characterized by emotional hypo- and hyper-reactivity. Soc Neurosci 8(2):136–147

Rizzolatti G, Griese F, Sinigaglia C (2008) Empathie und Spiegelneurone. Die biologische Basis des Mitgefühls. 1. Aufl. Suhrkamp, Frankfurt am Main (Edition Unseld, 11)

Schmeichel BJ, Demaree HA (2010) Working memory capacity and spontaneous emotion regulation: high capacity predicts self-enhancement in response to negative feedback. Emotion 10(5):739–744

Schmeichel BJ, Volokhov RN, Demaree HA (2008) Working memory capacity and the self-regulation of emotional expression and experience. J Pers Soc Psychol 95(6):1526–1540

Sullenberger C, Zaslow J (2009) Man muss kein Held sein. Auf welche Werte es im Leben ankommt. 1. Aufl. Bertelsmann, München

van Heijnsbergen CCRJ, Meeren HKM, Grèzes J, de Gelder B (2007) Rapid detection of fear in body expressions, an ERP study. Brain Res 1186:233–241

Wicker B, Keysers C, Plailly J, Royet JP, Gallese V, Rizzolatti G (2003) Both of us disgusted in my insula: the common neural basis of seeing and feeling disgust. Neuron 40(3):655–664

Successful Strategies to Detect and Avoid Failures

4

Eugen H. Bühle

Abstract

This chapter was written to point out the weakness of human beings in managing their tasks in a demanding situation. The higher the time pressure is, the more the stress level rises, and human beings tend to fail in managing their tasks.

This article shall give some hints to a start thinking in risk management categories under the specific aspect of the failure rate of human beings. The chapter shows different but statistically important human failures in complex environments. Even more important are the statements about reducing risks and so far reducing the human error rate.

Health industry is growing tremendously as human beings get older and older and new surgery techniques and medicinal drugs are implemented.

It is not an error to make an error once, but it is unbecoming of a doctor not to admit or to acknowledge his/her own error, thus making it impossible later to draw the necessary conclusions and to learn from the experience. (Georg Ernst Stahl (1660–1734) German doctor and chemist, physician to King Friedrich Wilhelm I of Prussia and Elector of Brandenburg)

4.1 Human Errors in the Medical Environment

Everybody knows how complex human beings are and therefore everybody understands that it is only human to make mistakes. Of course, the number of errors differs from person to person as we are individuals who are influenced by a variety of different factors. Naturally, we do not want to accept that this is true, but instinctively we know that we are object to a wide range of internal and external influencing factors.

E.H. Bühle
Bühle hpm-consult GmbH, Human performance management, Leitenhöhe 10, Herrsching 82211, Germany
e-mail: eugen.buehle@gmx.de

© Springer-Verlag Berlin Heidelberg 2016
W. Merkle (ed.), *Risk Management in Medicine*, DOI 10.1007/978-3-662-47407-5_4

Here is a brief overview of some of the factors which can influence our individual performance and thus have an effect on the number of errors we make:

- Fatigue
- Dullness/Lack of enthusiasm
- Ambience
- Working atmosphere
- Weather
- Stress
- Disturbances
- Rules which are not understood
- Procedures which are not understood
- Deviation from standard procedures
- Unsure process management
- Lack of time
- Individual motivation 'how we feel on the day'
- Lack of coordination within the team
- Conflict between team members
- Personal trouble
- Conflict with the boss
- Inadequate working environment and many others

4.1.1 Errors and Error Research

An error is a deviation from a defined norm which has been optimised in status and function in a determined system. In general an error is defined as a deviation from accuracy and correctness generally resulting in a deficiency. The *German Institute for Standardisation defines an error* as a value which is not reached by the requirements for a specific task. The occurrence of errors in general is an indication of a deficiency, and each error has specific consequences depending on its nature. Errors are usually classified according to the severity of their consequences.

The term *error culture* is known from the social and economic sciences where it refers to the way in which social systems deal with error risks, errors and the consequences of errors.

Human error research conducted at the end of the twentieth century focused on two main points.

In the early stages of error research, in times of growing industrialisation, attention was concentrated on errors originating from machines and devices, with a view to eliminating technical mistakes. As this research progressed and more and more experience was gathered particularly in the field of occupational psychology, scientists came to focus their attention on human beings as a major factor in the incidence of errors. The term *human factors* was introduced, under which we understand the susceptibility of human beings to making mistakes. The objective at that time was to increase productivity and to improve safety at work for the employees.

In the industrial world, as well as in hospitals (but here much later than in industry), the concept of 'quality management' was installed to deal with errors and to avoid errors in procedures and services.

In hospitals errors in treatment are to be found in anamnesis, diagnosis, therapy, surgery, postoperative treatment and inappropriate medication. This is by no means an exhaustive list, and there are many more error possibilities; the unfortunate truth is that where human beings are in action, errors will occur (Chap. 1).

4.1.2 General Consequences of an Error in Medical Treatment

According to official statements of several organisations concerned with patients' safety, a very high number of patients each year are victims of inappropriate medical treatment. The official numbers from the year 2013 are between 40,000 and 44,000. The real number is expected to be higher. About 17,000 patients die each year after treatment in a hospital as a result of avoidable medical errors.

The consequences of an error in medical treatment can be fatal for the patient, doctor and hospital (see Fig. 4.1).

- There is a possibility that the patient has to undergo another, more severe treatment or

Fig. 4.1 Lost clamp intraoperatively

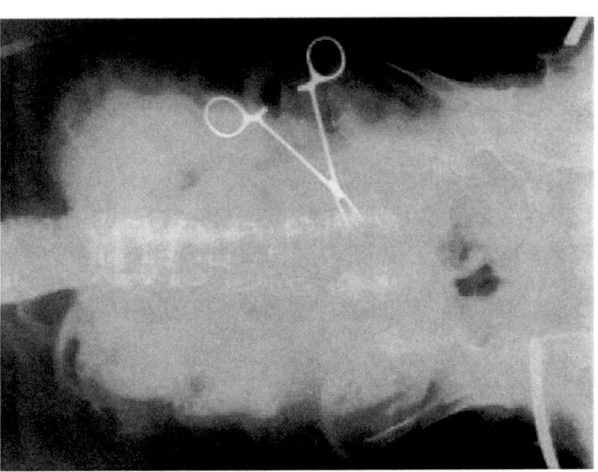

even additional surgery. In any case the overall duration of the treatment is prolonged. The worst-case scenario is when the additional treatment is not successful and the patient suffers lasting disability or even dies.

- The doctor who is responsible for the error (and for the patient) has to live with these consequences and in the worst event has to come to terms psychologically with the death of his/her patient. Patients have meanwhile become well organised and so there is a chance that after a medical error occurs, the patient looks for legal help. In recent years the rights of patients have been strengthened. In Germany, a new law, known as PRG (Patientenrechtegesetz = law governing patients' rights) came into force in 2013.

One fact which is quite certain in any case is that the health-care system has to bear the additional costs of the 'error treatment'. These expenses constitute a significant proportion of the total costs of the medical system.

The avoidance of errors in treatment indeed has positive effects for patients, the doctor and, of course, the health-care system. Hospitals as well will profit from fewer medical errors, as the additional expenses are reduced and this ultimately has an effect on health insurance premiums.

Thus, the goal of each medical treatment must be to avoid errors so that the patient, the doctor and the whole health-care system will benefit.

In the year 2012, the medical insurance services (MDK) carried out an assessment of medical errors in which the experts reviewed 12,483 notified medical errors. They found 3932 medical errors in hospitals and medical practices. This means that 30.5 % of all cases were found to be medical errors, and in 25 % of these cases, the error in medical treatment led directly to a health defect (see Chap. 2).

Two-thirds of the incidents were found in hospitals, and one-third was found in medical practices. Most of the errors occurred in the therapy of knee joints and hip joints. In most cases complaints were levelled at surgeons and orthopaedic doctors.

From these 12,483 cases, 3872 cases were from outpatient treatment of which 36 % were found as confirmed errors. 8607 cases were from treatment in hospitals with 29.5 % confirmed errors. This means that there were more than twice as many reported cases in hospitals as in outpatient treatment, but the percentage of treatments with an error was lower in hospitals.

Most of the confirmed accusations in outpatient treatments were found in dentistry including mouth and face surgery with an error rate of 49 %; gynaecology followed with 37.6 %

accusations and thereafter general medicine with 36.9 %.

In hospital units, the confirmed medical malpractice is found in nursing with 59 %, in neurosurgery with 31 %, gynaecology and midwifery with 29.6 % and anaesthesia and intensive medicine with 29.4 %.

The main concern of the medical statistics unit is the high number of confirmed errors in dentistry including mouth and face surgery, gynaecology, orthopaedics, casualty surgery and nursing with 58.9 % of all cases.

The general problem with the statistics is that only a fraction of the total number of cases of medical error is recorded. In Germany in the first quarter of 2011, about 45 million treatments were administered by doctors with more than 105 million contacts between patient and doctor as well as more than 16 million stationary hospital treatments. It is quite understandable that the estimated number of unrecorded cases is way higher.

Furthermore errors in internal medicine cases are more difficult to detect comparable to surgical disciplines and therefore more often overlooked.

4.1.3 Consequences of Errors for Patient, Doctor and Health-Care System

To deal properly with error management, of course, takes a certain time, but it seems to be absolutely necessary in order to avoid serious consequences for patients, doctors and the health-care system. It is equally desirable that the reputation of a medical practice or a hospital should not be endangered as a consequence of medical errors. A good reputation is of utmost importance if one is to retain one's patients and, even more so, to increase their numbers as this is a key factor in the economic scheme. If a reputation is lost because of medical errors, the practice or hospital will face economic consequences and it will be very difficult to regain confidence and rebuild a good reputation. In this context there is a great deal of truth in the axiom that 'Quality pays for itself'.

At the beginning of the 1990s, Gordon Guyatt coined the term 'evidence-based medicine' by which we understand the following: for each course of treatment planned, it is necessary to decide in the interest of the patient on the basis of empirically proven effectiveness. With this new way of thinking, the medical profession is trying to reduce the total rate of medical errors.

This approach certainly holds some potential for conflict in a framework which demands greater economic efficiency; health insurance companies are increasingly calling for (and are only prepared to pay for) treatments based on evidence of efficacy (evidence-based medicine). In all honesty, it must be pointed out that a very small proportion of the medical treatments being applied today are actually based on hard evidence.

The problems of this approach are therefore quite obvious, and in some individual cases the approach may be entirely unhelpful; evidence criteria certainly make sense for the majority of patients and cases, but not always. Sometimes there are individual particularities and it is possible to deviate from these criteria. Both the health insurers and the courts are aware of this. A precondition here, though, is that carefully maintained records must be kept to indicate why the medical practitioner chose to, or indeed had to, deviate from the guidelines.

4.2 Strategies to Avoid Errors

If one thinks about the consequences of medical errors, there should be only one solution for a doctor: the avoidance of errors must have absolute priority. After a successful medical treatment without any mishaps, the patient is happy and will come back when he/she has another health problem. If a medical error occurs, doctors and nurses have to invest further time and money in planning and providing treatment to correct this error. Nowadays, more than ever before, if errors have occurred, patients are likely to voice their criticism of doctors and/or hospitals in conversation with other potential patients. This naturally has an influence on the reputations concerned, and a loss of reputation means a loss of patients and, therefore, a loss of income.

If there were fewer errors in medical treatment, the whole health-care system would save a huge amount of money and would be way more efficient. The consequence would be that everyone would have to pay less for their medical insurance.

There are some strategies which ought to be observed in practices and hospitals to help to avoid errors. The possibilities of error avoidance are listed below, beginning with the so-called *human error*.

4.2.1 Swiss Cheese Model

In 1990 James Reason published his/her book *Human Error* and successfully implemented a new theory in the research of human susceptibility to making errors. His/her theory about the human factor is now a standard approach in human-error research. In the meantime, what he/she calls the 'Swiss cheese model' – for understanding how an error or failure can be avoided – has become a synonym among human-error experts for the concept of error avoidance.

Each slice of cheese represents a possibility for error defence. This layer of error defence could be the responsibility of the organisation, the management, the working environment, the team itself or any team member. Each slice has one or more holes, like the cheese, which represent the basic error risk faced by each work unit.

This potential for errors within any system is described as the latent conditions/failures. The latent errors in medicine could be: inadequate background information, wrong medication, missing or wrong results, personnel not qualified in accordance with requirements, doctor under excessive stress, etc.

If an error is made in each layer of defence (error illustrated symbolically by a hole in each slice of cheese), there will be a catastrophic outcome for the patient, as the error (arrow) will pass through all the layers without being noticed. By moving only one slice in the defence layer so that the error cannot pass through unnoticed, a potentially fatal mistake with all its accompanying consequences could be prevented (Fig. 4.2).

Knowing this, each person involved in the process of patient treatment should identify the error potential in his/her particular area and should devise appropriate countermeasures to prevent such errors.

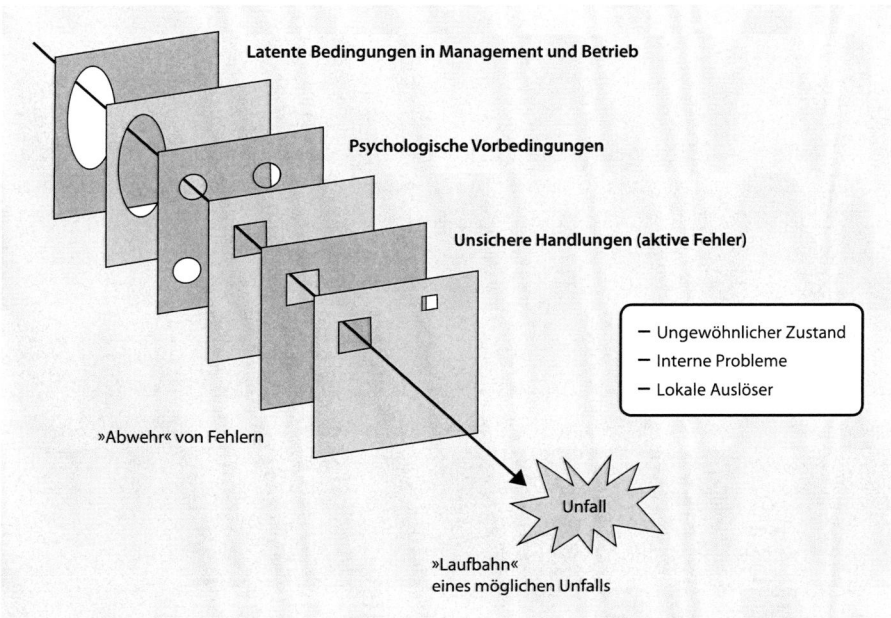

Fig. 4.2 Swiss Cheese Model

Each person should check and keep a critical eye on anyone involved in the process, not in order to criticise but to recognise the beginning of an error. Everyone has benefitted from having his/her attention drawn to a potential mistake in good time to enable it to be prevented; this is indeed one of the advantages of working in a team.

This approach reduces the probability of making errors. If an error occurs despite all the precautions, which is always likely to be the case, each person involved in the process should know how to handle the error and how to correct it. There should always be a plan B; if the wrong medication has been administered, the antidote should be known and immediately applied.

4.2.2 Process and Process Management

Process management in a hospital is of utmost importance even at the very beginning. A process can be described as clearly determined steps and clearly defined tasks which are the underpinning elements to achieve a specific goal.

A distinction is made between material processes, work processes, service processes, management processes and surgery processes. All of these processes are to be found in a medical practice as well as in a hospital; they are integrated in the system, and in many cases it is difficult to differentiate between them.

If we have a look, first of all, at the work processes, we can understand that by optimisation the efficiency can be improved and thus the error rate can be reduced as well. It is easy to see that greater efficiency and fewer errors have a direct correlation to cost and profit.

Errors often begin at the first contact with the patient during the registration and administration process and the documentation of the pathogenesis (Chap. 15). It is self-evident that all employees should have undergone specific training to know and to master all the processes within their area of responsibility. In line with the concept of delegation and responsibility, they should also have the authorisation to take decisions in their specified area.

To avoid errors, each doctor in a medical practice or hospital should periodically review the internal processes to adjust and manage them in a better way. In this context, *process management* means to optimise procedures in a closed loop.

Processes in a practice and in a hospital, especially in the operating theatre, can be extremely complex. Consequently, the first step in error prevention must be a thorough process analysis. For this to be successful, it is important that the head of the department and all the team members work together honestly and with an open mind. In many cases it might be more effective to involve an external consultant who is a process expert. Being from outside, this person can see things from a different perspective and may thus be able to judge more objectively.

Every single step in a process must be recorded and checked in terms of its necessity and efficacy. Process experts work with a specified matrix with which they analyse and assess every step in a course of action.

Of utmost importance is that everybody who is involved in the process, regardless of his/her hierarchical position, should take an active part in the analysis and in any subsequent change and optimisation.

In a workshop situation, it is the duty of the team leader/facilitator to find solutions in an open discussion about the optimisation of the process. This is a difficult task as in such teams specific traits of human behaviour tend to prevail. Staff members are not keen to change their opinions and positions and the processes they have become used to. With the help of an experienced external expert, it is easier to deal with these psychological phenomena (see Chap. 13).

4.2.3 Documentation of the Course of the Illness

In the process of medical treatment, we often tend to underestimate the significance of anamnesis, diagnosis and the *documentation* of the steps of the treatment.

Only unambiguous, clear and explicit documentation of the individual steps of the treatment carried out together with the positive and negative changes in the patient's condition enables the doctor to obtain an overall picture even at a later stage. Such a record may also serve as a basis for the successful creation of a later complaint or lawsuit by the patient (Chap. 15).

A form of documentation like this is helpful in long-lasting illnesses in that it provides an overview of the entire development of the illness and its symptoms. If the doctor has the entire, precisely documented overview, this makes it much easier for him/her to establish the course of the illness than fragments of documentation would.

In most cases in which it is claimed that medical errors have occurred, it is possible, on presentation of a particularly detailed record, to establish where, when and why the error happened during the medical treatment. At first, this seems to speak *against* keeping detailed documentation because in the event of an error, this information can be used against the doctor. But a detailed documentation is a strong argument in the context of error prevention because the whole history of the illness is recorded and any confusion or imprecision can be thus largely excluded. As is explained in detail in Chap. 15, a *lack of documentation* leads to a change in the burden of proof and perhaps even the loss of the legal case because activities that are not documented are considered 'not to have taken place'.

It is only with a thorough and detailed description of the symptoms of the illness and its treatment that it is possible to have a reliable measurement of the treatment's success or to find the causes of any failure. Carefully recorded documentation thus helps to identify and to prevent mistakes, to increase the success rate of patients treated and to avoid failures in any subsequent legal confrontations. It is difficult to imagine a better win-win situation.

4.2.4 Planning of Operations

It still happens today that many operations are performed 'on demand', which means that the surgeon has neither been previously concerned with the patient and his/her individual complaints nor is he/she mentally prepared for the task.

In such situations it is absolutely necessary to hold a meeting ('briefing' prior to the operation with all those participating in the operation to discuss the patient's condition and indications, to clarify the medical findings, to lay down the procedure to be followed and to assess the individual risks for this patient undergoing this operation). This discussion should make use of all the media that are available today (Chaps. 1, 6, 12 and 14).

The procedure should be guided by 'evidence-based models' and 'best-practice models'. For example, the way such a team meeting could be conducted can be found in Chap. 14.

The day before the operation, the surgeon should be intensively involved with the patient and with the background to his/her complaint so that he/she can form a 'mental model' of the forthcoming surgical intervention. What is meant by a *mental model* is the forming of a mental image of the reality of the operation, defining the appropriate approach to be adopted and the techniques to be used. By using a 'mental model' in the preparation of a complex operation, the likelihood of errors occurring can be drastically reduced. This is the experience gained in the aviation field and in top-level competitive sport which, without these psychological aids, would not be in a position to provide the safety standard or the performances achieved.

4.2.5 Standardised Procedures and Rules

The standards and rules applied within an organisation make a major contribution to assuring smooth coordination and quality within that organisation. Standards are recognised procedures promoting conformity which have empirically proved their ability to fulfil the demands of the situation. They provide the basis for coordinated action within processes which involve a number of individuals or teams.

When the objective is to prevent the occurrence of mistakes, the main priority in doctor's practices as well as in hospitals should be to define, and consistently maintain, standard procedures and processes. This also means that there should be a standardised set of operating instruments assigned to every surgical procedure. As a rule, individual approaches and individual sets of instruments are to be discouraged.

The best approach is for the senior physician in a practice or the senior consultant in a hospital to define the standards in collaboration with the members of staff, and these are to be implemented in rules which are binding on all participants (known as *SOP*, *s*tandard *o*peration *p*rocedures).

This also requires a significant amount of work and effort, but this pays off in the broadest sense of the word in the reduction in the incidence of mistakes. Verbal definitions or regulations, however, are only a partial achievement because after only a short time, differences in interpretation and processes start to creep in. For this reason procedures and rules have to be laid down in writing.

4.2.6 Handbook

A handbook can be used for the documentation of procedures and rules where all participants can read them and understand them. In order to avoid misunderstandings and subsequent mistakes, the duties within a team must be clearly and unambiguously assigned and defined. The head of the department must make it quite clear that the person responsible for a task also assumes responsibility for correct implementation. When necessary, if the head of department deviates from these defined rules, he/she must also accept that the person responsible for applying the rules should remind him/her that they must be observed.

In medical practices or hospital departments, these standard procedures together with a description of duties are best laid down in a handbook in which the details of the procedures must be described precisely. Each member of the team must be in possession of a copy of such a handbook; as a rule nowadays, such handbooks are in electronic form so that all the people concerned have access to them easily.

The person responsible for the handbook must update it at regular intervals. The current version is to be documented and old versions must be removed or deleted.

The handbook is a great help to new people joining the team and in particular those completing their training, enabling them to settle in quickly and to understand the in-house procedures and the distribution of duties.

4.2.7 Communication

In the context of the avoidance of errors, communication has a highly significant role to play. Clear and unambiguous communication helps to avoid misunderstandings. Misunderstandings are often the cause of mistakes. This applies to treatments carried out in doctors' practices but much more so to surgical interventions in an operating theatre (Chap. 10).

It must be completely clear to the operating team before the operation what the surgical intervention will be and where the particular risks lie. If there are to be deviations from standard procedures, all the participants must be given detailed information beforehand and the approach and procedure to be adopted must be clearly presented.

In particular when complications arise, quick and safe action is demanded. The doctor responsible then has the duty to inform all the members of the staff of the measures to be taken and to issue clear, unambiguous and personally assigned instructions. The important thing here is that the person who holds overall responsibility should ask the opinions of the staff and to take these into consideration in his/her deliberations (Chaps. 1 and 6).

4.2.8 Sequential Briefing

'Talk your doing' is what the Americans say and, in this way, triggers a thought process among those involved in the activity.

This procedure is used in aviation and, by virtue of a remark from an accompanying colleague/

observer, has already on many occasions prevented errors with possibly risky consequences. In the aviation sector, this procedure is known as *sequential briefing*.

During a surgical intervention, the operating surgeon should speak about every new action beforehand and make it transparent what he/she is going to do next and how he/she intends to do it. This approach is new and, at first, is difficult to put into practice but offers another possibility to avert mistakes before they arise. As a rule, successful surgeons often proceed in this way quite intuitively.

By making actions transparent, the active surgeon is obliged, before taking a step, to describe the step and thus to think it through again before taking action; the assistant is also required to go through the steps in his/her 'mental model' and to compare and assess them. If his/her understanding of the procedure is different, he/she must say so and give an appropriate indication (Chaps. 1 and 6).

4.2.9   Reviewing and Checking

An important procedure for preventing mistakes consists of breaking down the work process into its individual steps.

After completion of every step of the operation, the step is checked to ensure that the action was performed correctly and without mistakes. A good example of such an action could be the checking of the stitching of the large intestine and the subsequent positioning of the intestine in the abdominal cavity before the next step, the closing of the abdominal wall, begins; the usual counting of the abdominal layers before the closure of the wound is also one of these checking measures.

This all takes time and 'time is money'. But this is a short-sighted perspective, as the following example shows: if the surgeons performing an operation on the large intestine had proceeded in this way, they would have noticed the failure to stitch up the large intestine and would have corrected the error. As it happened, their attention was drawn to the omission only days later when the patient complained of severe abdominal

pains. The comments from the doctors concerned that 'pain is part of the healing process' merely served to delay even further the search for the causes and, after a few more days' waiting, the abdomen had to be reopened in an emergency operation.

> **Example: Human Error** It happens still too often that scissors, clamps or even entire cloths are left inside the abdomen. Following a Caesarean section, a woman complained of severe pain and sought help at the hospital. Her anxieties were met with soothing words and she was sent home reassured. During that night she collapsed and her husband took her to the nearest hospital casualty department. Her abdomen was opened and a cloth appeared.
>
> Human error is quite inexcusable, but with absolute certainty it could have been avoided by careful review and checking measures (e.g. counting the number of cloths).

4.2.10 Checklists and Their Benefits

In the pioneering years of aviation, after numerous flying accidents had occurred as a result of mistakes in operation, checklists were introduced for individual phases of the flight. The philosophy behind this was that all actions, switching operations and preparatory measures should be completed before they are confirmed by reading the checklist. The reading of checklists is part of the standard procedure for pilots even though after many years of flying experience, they may know the procedures and checklists by heart. The reading of a checklist is a standard procedure which can be applied in all situations.

The WHO also recommends the introduction of checklists for operating theatres. Unfortunately, there is still considerable resistance to this, and there are far too few hospitals where checklists have become part of standard procedures.

It frequently happens that the wrong operating instruments were prepared or that various items of equipment did not function and were not checked by the staff prior to the operation. Such incidents can be eliminated by the use of checklists (Chap. 6).

We are all human and thus, even with many years of experience and established routine, are prone to making mistakes (see Human Error). Because this is the case, checklists can help to prevent omissions and subsequent errors.

> **Example: The Benefits of Checklists**
> Even after decades of aviation activity, checklists still provide the security that nothing has been forgotten, and despite the many years of experience, it can happen that the list occasionally draws the operator's attention to an omission.

4.2.11 Training

Learning by doing – it is still the case nowadays that junior doctors admit that the first wound they stitched was, in fact, on a patient, albeit under the watchful eyes of an experienced colleague.

It is still not a widespread habit to practice how to stitch up wounds using, e.g. pig intestines. The same applies to learning how to wield a scalpel. Practice using pieces of meat would help to prepare doctors for the 'real thing'. By contrast, with the increasingly widespread introduction of what is known as minimally invasive surgery, practice on a simulator is already very common to ensure that the doctor's first steps represent no danger for patients.

Three-dimensional images represented on computer screen and extended arms and fingers at the end of a mechanical structure present the operating surgeon with a particularly daunting challenge. Without practice and training before use of such equipment for a real operation, mistakes in laparoscopic surgery are practically preprogrammed.

The medical industry has recognised this and offers increasing opportunities to practice using a simulator. In the aviation field, simulation activities in a hi-fi flight simulator have been common practice worldwide since the 1960s for the teaching, exercising and training of pilots. A flight simulator recreates reality very authentically. Not only does it represent the normal flying conditions with movement, noise and visual images of the view from the cockpit but, for training purposes, it can also provide flying behaviour compatible with an emergency situation such as engine failure or the loss of the hydraulic system.

Every pilot is obliged to spend 4 h at least four times per year together with a certified trainer and coach in such a 'flight simulator device' and he/she must complete two examinations. Only in this way can the industry guarantee that in real life a captain and co-pilot acting as a team will deal with emergency situations reliably and professionally.

A security concept of this kind is widely foreign to the medical profession. Hopefully the very first concepts of OR simulators will be successful and lead to routine use in the future.

4.3 Contributing Factors Which Can Lead to Mistakes

A variety of factors contributing to mistakes are known from Human Factors research. The doctor is no exception here as he/she too is subject to human weaknesses and the associated susceptibility to making mistakes. In aircraft accident research, these factors are called the *contributing factors* which arise as a consequence of our human behaviour.

4.3.1 Laxness, Carelessness

Laxness and/or carelessness, known in aviation accident research as 'complacency', is one of the known factors. Pilots and doctors do not always act with the necessary care since routine has a soporific effect and leads over the years to a tendency to be lax or to act carelessly in familiar situations.

This also applies to anamnesis, medical treatment or surgical operations. Many things are merely regarded as pure routine and are handled laxly (because they are bothersome). The approach is to suppose that the task is routine, the behavioural ritual corresponds to this assessment, the result tends to be left to chance rather than being specifically planned and the unexpected soon occurs.

'Murphy's law' takes its name from the American engineer E.A. Murphy Jr. The law says that

Whatever can go wrong will go wrong.

Or, in other words,

If there is more than one possible outcome of a job or task, and one of the outcomes will result in disaster or an undesirable consequence, then somebody will do it that way.

From our own experience of life, we must all know that everything that can go awry inevitably does.

The best approach to prevent mistakes is thus to go about one's tasks with the greatest concentration and maintaining of all the standards and rules and with the attitude 'expect the unexpected'.

4.3.2 Overestimation of One's Own Abilities

In many accidents in civil aviation, the report comes to the conclusion that the 'probable cause' of the accident was the '*overconfidence* of the captain and lack of teamwork'.

What is to be understood by overconfidence is the misguided assessment of one's own abilities which tends to arise in most people after many years of routine work coupled with a lack of a self-critical faculty. People feel that they have already successfully mastered so many situations, so there is no reason why it should be different this time.

This is a typical example of overconfidence. If the specialised department had been informed in good time, the patient's life could have been saved.

Example: Overestimation of One's Own Abilities One example of this is when an experienced surgeon ventures to perform an operation which is not in his/her field of expertise and which would have been the task of specialists in another department. When complications arise, the surgeon believes he/she can master the situation and does not even ask his/her specialised colleagues to come to his/her assistance. The patient dies.

4.3.3   Tiredness

Tiredness is also one of the contributing factors, because when we are tired we cannot achieve our normal powers of concentration. Night-shift duties which are low staffed and place high demands on the doctor in the hospital or at the sight of an accident are particularly prone to this factor. This means that distinct tiredness resulting from a lack of sleep and/or work in opposition to the body's natural rhythms gives rise to a higher incidence of errors than work performed after a good night's sleep. What is more, when one is tired, one's own critical faculties no longer function properly – with the risk, e.g. of overconfidence (see above).

There is very little precautionary action that one can take in advance to combat tiredness during a night shift; with considerable self-discipline and maintaining regular breaks, it is possible to keep one's effective performance at a constant, albeit reduced, level (Chap. 6). The only effective precautionary measures are correct timetables of duty which regulate the physiologically necessary recuperation and sleep requirements. Periods of time on duty covering 72 h at a stretch, which were indeed quite common even until quite recently, must not be allowed to occur.

4.3.4   Alcohol

It is widely known that the excessive consumption of alcohol, with residual alcohol in the blood, has a deleterious effect on a person's performance.

There is good reason for the 0.5‰ limit for motorists, and there are a number of drivers whose abilities are already impaired at this level, i.e. they show a greater susceptibility to making mistakes, whereas there are other individuals who only begin to show this effect with double this amount of alcohol in the blood.

In the aviation world, the axiom is '12 hours from the bottle to the throttle', i.e. no alcohol within the 12 h prior to a flight/service, and, before that naturally, only in moderation. In my opinion this rule should also apply in the medical world, since here too people's lives are at stake. A conscientious doctor certainly acts responsibly with regard to his/her alcohol consumption.

4.3.5 Dealing with Stress

It is absolutely undisputed in occupational psychology that stress has an enormous effect on the quality of the work performed. Everybody has experienced this negative effect for him- or herself and knows that when you try to perform complex tasks under time pressure, together with the pressure to achieve, there is a drastic increase in the incidence of mistakes.

Each person responds to stressful situations quite differently. Not everyone manages to remain calm and composed, which would be helpful in order to prevent mistakes. 'Anti-stress seminars' would be of assistance here. However, they are not widely popular in the medical field.

Regular sport activity also helps to make unsuitably high stress levels more 'digestible' as well as being a prophylactic measure against stressful situations, which nowadays are a typical feature of the daily work of a doctor. However, the increasing burden of work seems to allow little time for regular sport. Yet it is well known that freedom and endurance sports help to 'clear the head' so that work activity that follows can be dealt with more efficiently and without errors. The time supposedly 'wasted' is thus quickly compensated for.

Further information about the additional risks accompanying an excessive workload for a doctor is to be found in the article entitled 'Burnout' published in the Hessischen Arzteblatt February 2013 (further details also on the LÄKH website).

4.3.6 Decision-Making

In a complex situation with unexpected findings and with a limited time available to act, decisions must be reached swiftly.

We know that in a situation with mounting stress, it is difficult to reach a structured decision. When under stress, people tend to take gut decisions which in general are possibly based on empirical reasons but which are not properly thought through in all their implications. In an unstructured decision-making process, the likelihood of making mistakes increases dramatically (Chaps. 1 and 6).

What is important is that before the decision is taken, the facts are clear and understood, and that the options for action are all examined.

Each of the possible courses of action must be evaluated in terms of its advantages and disadvantages. Discussion within the team can be helpful here in reaching a balanced decision after evaluation of all the foreseeable risks. The important thing is that the consequences of all the possible options are all thought through and assessed beforehand prior to reaching a decision to proceed in a particular way (Chap. 11).

4.4 Leadership and Management

In this context, the significance of the role played by the management of a practice or a hospital unit, and indeed the management of a hospital or clinic as a whole, has to be recognised, too. Part of the task of staff management is to ensure that the processes, the flow of information, the personal attention given to employees and the motivation engendered are designed appropriately by the administration forces. Regulations and expectations are to be formulated and the individual areas of responsibility are to be unambiguously defined.

Professional management of staff pays off because motivated employees perform better work and make fewer mistakes. The atmosphere in a practice or hospital has a major role to play here because the evidence shows that in a work environment with considerate, open and collegial behaviour, fewer mistakes occur. When employees are involved in the design of processes, their creativity and experience are put to use in bringing grievances to light, eliminating them and optimising processes.

In the process of making the medical service more economically efficient, professional personnel management seems to have restricted itself in many hospitals to the mere reduction of the workforce in order to reduce costs with the result that the remaining employees suffer under an even greater workload and there is no time at all to reflect on the way the work is performed – with the ultimate outcome that the incidence rate of mistakes increases. A serious rethink is absolutely necessary in this context.

4.4.1 Employee Suggestion Scheme

A progressive medical practice or hospital management is able to involve employees in the improvement of processes. This can also be achieved by the introduction of an internal suggestion scheme in which employees are invited to submit written proposals for improvements.

In such a hospital, a form is available to employees to make suggestions for improvements and to post them in a special postbox, e.g. in the operating unit. Once such a tool has been created, it is interesting to see how many suggestions are submitted which are then assessed by the body which is also responsible for their implementation. No hospital can really afford to ignore the potential that is latent in such a system.

The evaluation of suggestions must take place soon after submission, and feedback must be sent to the employee concerned with the results of the examination. The crucial part of the scheme is not the scarcity of suggestions but rather that these must be examined without any reservations

and, above all, that they are subsequently implemented and changes are put into effect by the doctors and hospital managers.

The potential that lies in suggestions made by employees who are directly involved in daily activities is enormous. Savings in work, time, materials and personnel involvement also serve to prevent mistakes. For such a suggestion scheme to be successful, there needs to be a reward system which has a motivating effect on employees. A scheme of this kind is still largely unknown in hospitals.

Some time ago in Japan, the concept of 'Kaizen' (which translates as 'change for the better') was introduced in the automotive industry. In well-managed, commercial enterprises, it has now become normal to talk of processes of continuous improvement. This frame of mind, which is constantly looking for and remedying weakness in processes, should also be introduced into our medical services with a view to optimising procedures and thus preventing mistakes (Chaps. 1 and 6).

4.4.2 The Doctor as the Boss and the Hierarchical Gradient

Naturally, the overall responsibility for the smooth running of operations in a medical practice lies with the doctor, with the senior consultant in a hospital unit or with the executive management in a hospital. They are the people who, by the way in which they manage their staff, set the atmosphere in the 'health business' and thus influence the incidence of mistakes. At first sight, the layperson would not find this understandable. Yet it had been scientifically shown that in a pleasant work environment, people make fewer mistakes than they make in a distinctly hierarchically structured environment where the tone is occasionally rather harsh (Chaps. 5 and 6).

Staff working under very dominant and authoritative senior consultants often does not have the courage to indicate deficiencies in processes and erroneous methods of treatment or they even shy away from seeking advice from the senior consultant. Staff members that are authoritatively managed and who dare not challenge this authority are afraid of making mistakes themselves and they tend to make mistakes. Such mistakes are then concealed as the person concerned is too afraid to own up to the error honestly and to deal with the situation. This is one of the reasons why an anonymous error-reporting system is one way of revealing mistakes without any sanctions (Chap. 9). In operating theatres that are run in this way, the only person who speaks is the senior consultant. Neither the assistant nor the operating-theatre nurses actively involve themselves in the operation but only respond to orders/requests given to them.

It is well known that the hierarchical structure in hospitals is still very pronounced. Yet it has been shown for some time that distinct hierarchies tend to suppress critical comments (from staff members) which are aimed at preventing errors. This means, in turn, in order to prevent mistakes, that it makes sense to encourage staff members to give careful thought to what they are doing and to voice their opinions. In such hospitals employees do not dare to point out a mistake to the senior consultant, even less to make a suggestion.

The solution lies in designing flatter hierarchies which involve staff in all the procedures and which take their opinions into consideration. This approach of itself is a way of showing respect and appreciation and helps to create an atmosphere of mutual trust and to reduce the distance between people.

4.4.3   Social Competence

In such hospitals specialist registrars, assistants, operating-theatre nurses, the nursing staff in general and, of course, the patients all complain off the record about the senior consultant's behaviour.

A study conducted in a reputable airline company revealed that the majority of the incidents endangering safety arose from the combination of operational problems, errors by pilots and problems resulting from social interactions. It seems evident then that the rate of mistakes could be reduced if people had the appropriate social skills. The training provided by reputable airlines quite deliberately trains their captains in the social skills necessary with a view to reducing the incidence of errors (Chap. 5).

4.4.4   The Organisation and the Management of Staff Members

Similarly, with regard to this subject, the management executives of a hospital cannot escape their responsibility because they are the ones who shape the working atmosphere in their hospital enterprise. It is also widely known that in a bad working atmosphere, the commitment of the employees is limited and so the result of the work performed leaves something to be desired. Open and honest communication on the part of the management of the hospital in its dealings with the works council and the employees is a precondition for responsible social interaction.

Since it is becoming more common for hospitals to be privatised, the management naturally is placed under considerable pressure to be financially efficient. In many cases this pressure is cascaded down the hierarchy so that everyone suffers from it.

Example: Discussion with Employee
A hospital doctor reported that by the end of May he/she had increased his/her performance by 15 % vis-à-vis the previous year. When he/she was called to meet the board of management, he/she expected his/her and his/her team's outstanding performance to be recognised. Far from it, the management board was of the opinion that if an increase of 15 % could be achieved in 6 months, it could assume that this would be doubled in the following 6 months. This doctor never entered into contact willingly with the management again and was no longer motivated to achieve any further increase in the number of cases he/she dealt with.

Among the leadership tasks incumbent on the management are also those related to the staff such as planning, communication of information, transparency, organisation, problem solution, motivation, consultation, development, further training, conflict resolution, recognition, appreciation, process design, monitoring, etc.

Particularly important is the management duty in conjunction with changes within the organisation. Change management is a real challenge and needs experienced managers who are able to gain the involvement and enthusiasm of the employees in the process of change. If a hospital is facing complex changes, it is often advisable to seek the assistance of an external expert (see Chap. 11).

4.5 Ways of Recognising Mistakes

Fatal errors are often first noticed when it is no longer possible to repair them 100 %. Often evidence of an error appears only days or weeks later when the patient complains of pain. What is crucially important in such cases is that efforts must be made to find the cause of the pain and the symptoms the patient complains of. It is always good to keep Murphy's law in mind, particularly when one believes that everything was done properly during the preceding operation/medical treatment.

4.5.1 Awareness of the Situation

Anyone who deals responsibly with the possibilities that medicine offers must be fully aware of the implications and consequences of the situation every time technical aids are used or every time there is surgical intervention. This means that it must be clear from the outset how to proceed, what tools and equipment are going to be used and what risks are involved. Adequate provision must be made in terms of the time necessary, together with a suitable additional safety margin, because the general tendency is to plan too little time rather than too much. This must

also apply in times of so-called optimised surgical operation planning with a high efficiency of theatre use and rapid changeover times.

It is important that staff members should work with higher concentration and that the stress level is kept at an appropriately low level. Time pressure translates directly into stress. It must be clear at all times at what stage in the process one finds oneself, what has already been done and what remains to be done. Decisions that have to be made must be soundly reasoned, clearly structured and readily understandable to everyone.

The consequences of each step of a course of action must be checked beforehand (Chap. 11), and if there are doubts about the outcome, alternatives should be examined. If, despite these precautions, a mistake occurs, the consequences must be quickly assessed and corrective measures taken. When people work with a very pronounced awareness of the situation, the potential for mistakes is already recognised in advance. Accordingly, the number of mistakes can be considerably reduced.

4.5.2 Teamwork

Intensive teamwork helps to prevent mistakes occurring because when people really work together closely, they communicate with each other. It must be quite clear to each team member what is going on. Before surgical intervention takes place, there must have been a meeting to discuss the case (Chap. 6). Yet communication must take place not only before but also during the operation. As already mentioned, the planned procedure must be referred to and the implementation must be commented upon (Chap. 10).

If this approach is adopted, the assistant or the theatre nurse is given the opportunity to voice concerns and, as appropriate, to make critical comments or refer to corrective measures. The voicing of concerns is not intended in the sense of criticism but rather as a mutually supportive measure. From our experience we know that, initially, a senior consultant finds it difficult if critical comments are made by the team. If there is no trusting relationship between the parties and staff members are not encouraged to become involved and to voice criticism, it is unlikely that any criticism will ever be heard.

If the senior consultant expresses thanks for the ideas and comments contributed, the initial natural reserve on the part of the team members can quickly be transformed, and one can be sure that before a serious mistake is made, attention will be drawn to it by one of the team members.

4.6   Handling Mistakes and Mistake Culture

Human beings, no matter how well prepared they are, are naturally not infallible, and consequently, mistakes will occur. We have to learn to deal with this situation. It is important that we should try to remain objective. It is ultimately inexpedient and unhelpful to cover up mistakes, so this should be avoided.

If a mistake occurs, it is important and correct to own up to it, to mention it immediately and to correct it. Here it must be remembered that corrective measures should also be carefully thought through in order not to compound the situation with further mistakes. This is best done within a team. If the team has failed to prevent the mistake, it will be that much more motivated to ensure that it is corrected properly.

The culture of blame in hospitals should thus be a thing of the past (Chap. 1).

4.6.1   Learning from Mistakes

People do not like to admit mistakes and are prepared even less to come to grips with clearly evident mistakes – they make the vow never to make the same mistake again. With a view to promoting a 'no blame' culture with regard to mistakes in medical practices and hospitals, it is essential to adopt a consistent approach to the correction of mistakes.

Every time people try to come to grips with their mistakes, this provides an opportunity to build on the insights gained and to learn and improve and thus to prevent this or similar mistakes again (Kaizen). When tackling mistakes, it is important that an attempt is made to identify the causes that led to the error. If the cause is defined, then a procedure or a work process can be developed to avoid mistakes with the same cause. This thought process is the basis for the CIRS method (Chaps. 1 and 9).

4.6.2   Share Your Experience

To promote a beneficial process of experience sharing, it is particularly important to tell colleagues about the experience you gained from a mistake situation. There are many ways of doing this. It must be seen as a major step towards error prevention if mistakes made within a department, a hospital or a medical practice are discussed internally and ways are found of preventing such mistakes in the future. Meetings of this kind are held far too seldom, mostly for the common reasons of a lack of time and money.

But this is to overlook the fact that mistakes cost money. A correct calculation of the costs arising from a mistake or, similarly, the costs of preventing a mistake must take account of the potential human suffering that can be avoided by the prevention of mistakes in medical treatment. In the light of such a comprehensive calculation, it would be clear that error prevention is cost-effective (Chaps. 19 and 20).

The establishment of a culture of learning from mistakes requires openness and honesty on the part of all the people concerned in their dealings with each other and in confrontations with the technical and non-personal aspects of their work. For the purpose of dealing with mistakes, there must be a possibility to publish an internally distributed document produced by a quality management body for the employees.

4.6.3   Critical Incident Reporting System (CIRS)

It is quite normal practice for airlines to report not only on errors within their own flight operations but also on incidents with other airlines.

A safety department accountable to the management board is responsible for evaluating such incident reports.

Incidents are registered with the safety department either anonymously or with a name. After the incidents have been evaluated by the department's specialists, the reports, official statements and opinions are published and made available to all pilots. Experience shows that these reports are read avidly and every pilot studies each situation described very intensively to ensure that in his/her own activities he/she does not make the same mistake.

This approach is very seldom seen in the medical field. It has been pioneered in urology with the book series entitled *Complications in Urology*. Three volumes have been published so far and they focus primarily on errors occurring in surgical interventions. These cases are evaluated, the causes are sought and better solution options are proposed for similar cases.

In the aviation field, if the errors are to be found in processes in the technical, clearance or flight procedures, a task force is set up which then, after studying all the details, introduces changes in the processes or flight procedures as necessary. The aircraft manufacturers, too, are involved in the search for a solution so that, by making modifications, similar or the same mistakes can be avoided in the future.

If the CIRS systems, currently being introduced to many hospitals, existed all over the country, a considerable number of mistakes could be excluded from the outset This would also mean that the consequences of mistakes, such as the additional costs and the supplementary work, would also be avoided and patients spared a great deal of suffering.

For details see Chap. 11.

4.7   Concluding Remarks

'All theory is grey' if you do not put it into practice. In further medical training, 99 % of the courses focus on medical subjects. The necessity for this is undisputed, but other subjects such as risk and error management, communication, teamwork etc., should also be included in training programmes in the future.

Personnel management skills are only rarely among today's criteria for recruitment in the medical field. In a renowned airline company, a pilot who was unable to display such abilities when examined and selected would never become a captain. Deficiencies in social competence when dealing with patients and staff in particular are noticeable in many cases. A lack of social competence tends to be conducive to the occurrence of errors.

This deficiency is primarily a failure of management; upper echelons of management must feel it their obligation to develop and improve the doctor's expertise also in the field of staff leadership and management; current advertisements emphasise above all the medical and economic skills of prospective senior consultants. Seminars focusing on the subject of personnel leadership/management should be offered to doctors and should be attended by them (see Chap. 7).

Nevertheless, we must not forget that, despite all the justified criticism of the current lack of error management systems in the medical profession and in hospitals, the overwhelming majority of patients receive highly competent personal and medical treatment. Yet, the mission 'nihil nocere' must still apply, and risk management must become an integral part of everyday medical practice, too.

From Theory to Practice: Risk Management in Hands-On Flight Operations

5

Dieter Hensel and Cord-H. Becker

Abstract

At first glance, risk management, as presented in the field of medicine, seems to be far removed from aviation. This is very shortsighted.

We will analyze how important it is to follow certain rules to improve safety; we believe that the following characteristics are essential:

A high degree of discipline, open communication, a perception of low hierarchy, decisions which always favor safety, and a relaxed approach to teamwork.

Today we know that the human factor can be the cause of incidents and accidents in the aviation business....

By using several examples of aircraft accidents, we would like to demonstrate the complexity of pilots' work in the cockpit and the link between little mistakes one can make and their possibly fatal consequences in aviation business. Medical parallels are pointed out following the aviation examples thus learning process could be supported.

At first glance, risk management, as presented in the field of medicine, seems to be far removed from aviation. This is very shortsighted. As presented in Chap. 1, we know which principles underlie risk management processes so that analogies between medicine and aviation are not far removed from one another; in aviation applied risk management is the basis for safety. There are important lessons to be learned here. The following text serves this purpose.

5.1 Introduction

To get from point A to point B, the safest way is, without a doubt, flying in an airplane. At the same time, we all know that airplanes do not escape accidents, sometimes, unfortunately, with deadly results.

In order to judge which method of travel is the safest, we must compare airplanes, trains, ships, automobiles, and other vehicles. When the number of travelers is compared to the number of

---

D. Hensel, MD (✉)
ATS Aviation Training Services,
Leibnizring 13, Kriftel 65830, Germany
e-mail: dieter.hensel@web.de

C.-H. Becker
ATS Aviation Training Support,
Gustav-Freytag-Str. 15, Wiesbaden 65189, Germany
e-mail: cord@cordbecker.de

© Springer-Verlag Berlin Heidelberg 2016
W. Merkle (ed.), *Risk Management in Medicine*, DOI 10.1007/978-3-662-47407-5_5

those injured or even to the number of fatalities, the airplane is always evaluated as the safest mode of travel.

5.2   Influences on Safe Flight Operations

The environment in which we fly is fragile and subject to many differing elements. These include to a large extent weather conditions such as rain, thunderstorms, snowfall, strong winds, wind shear, turbulence, icing, hale, lightning, fog, or even volcanic eruptions with ensuing ash clouds.

Additionally, there are laws of physics which influence every flight, such as the weight of the plane, engine performance, aerodynamic limits, runway texture, airport elevation, and surrounding airport topography. Also typical route criteria for areas such as the polar region, equator, and intertropical convergence zones play a role.

Very important factors include aircraft technology, the performance of air traffic control, the quality of aircraft maintenance, and especially the human factor; in this case, we, the pilots, exert a direct influence on flight safety.

5.3   Criteria in Flight Operations

To ensure success, each flight operation must orient itself to the following criteria: safety, economic efficiency, punctuality, passenger comfort, and environmental sustainability. Among these, safety must always be primary – as the saying goes, safety first! The strategy of error prevention plays a key role in our workplace.

Which strategies of error prevention help us to realize safe flight operations? Without wanting to suggest a ranking of importance, we believe that the following characteristics are essential:

A high degree of discipline in following procedures
Open communication
A perception of low hierarchy in the crew
Decisions which always favor safety
A relaxed approach to teamwork

A high level of expertise is not only required for flying skills. Competence and authority become apparent in a team-oriented leadership style.

It may sound simple but it's important nonetheless:

Four eyes see more than two.
Four ears hear more than two.
Two heads think more than one.

This means that team-thinking automatically creates human redundancy.

5.4   The Profile of Requirements for Cockpit Crews

In any discussion of tolerance, teamwork, and open communication, it is always the captain who remains solely responsible for each flight, and this is without restriction.

Among the so-called soft skills are for us:

- Willingness to take over responsibility
- Ability to be part of a team
- Leadership ability
- But also risk minimization

All of these skills are essential requirements for pilots.

What is noticeable among the findings of aircraft accidents is that the "human factor" accounts for more than 50 % of all accidents. At one time, one spoke of pilot error. Today we know that the human factor in other areas can be the cause of airplane accidents. These can be mistakes made by air traffic control, mistakes by maintenance, mistakes in computer development, or even mistakes in construction.

5.5   Risk Management of an Airline

The environment of the aviation industry, or as one says today "aviation business," is changing rapidly. Based on our own experience, we know that our pilot colleagues, hired as young pilots by the new Lufthansa in 1955, were able to end their careers as Jumbo captains. These colleagues experienced a quantum leap in the technical development of their aircraft – from the Fieseler Storch to the Boeing 747.

Of course this technical development is continuing rapidly. In contrast, the profile of requirements and the characteristics of a discretionary pilot selection remain unchanged in many important segments. Every applicant must display good spatial perception skills, technical understanding, psychomotor skills, as well as the ability to withstand stress in order to successfully practice this occupation. Having good grades is not a top priority. Rather, it is the abovementioned abilities which must always be present in order to operate an aircraft. Of course good grades in the core subjects of German, English, mathematics, and physics are important. What is crucial is that the test results in all subjects are above average. Deficiency in spatial perception cannot, for example, be balanced out with better results in mathematics.

This is the reason why the success rate of pilot selection lies between 5 and 10 %.

By using several examples, we would like to demonstrate the complexity of operating sequences in the cockpit and the link that little mistakes can make to their possibly fatal consequences.

We do not have the right to point our finger at others. After an accident, hindsight is always 20/20. The following cases have actually occurred.

5.6   Technical Inspections According to the Manual

After a successful technical inspection of an Airbus in Toulouse, the customer airline requested an additional "run-up" (engine test). The brakes were set, and the engine power was increased to maximum thrust. At this point, the plane began to skid forwards towards a wall. The thrust was greater than the power of the brakes which was to hold the aircraft in place. Attempts to stop the

plane by engaging the brake several times in the cockpit were ineffective. As the plane continued to move forwards, the fuselage was pressed upwards against the wall, resulting in a total loss of the aircraft. No one in the cockpit even considered pulling back on the thrust levers to reduce the engine power. For this particular test run, there was no defined procedure and no checklist. Luckily, no one was hurt. The damage: 180 million US dollars.

The conclusion: Do not "stick" to checklists but consider every angle in unusual situations.

5.7   Tailstrike

During takeoff in Melbourne for a flight to Dubai, the thrust was insufficient to lift the aircraft off the ground. At the point of rotation when the aircraft is to lift off, the tail section dragged along the runway. The aircraft lifted off too late, overrunning the end of the runway. The aircraft suffered major structural damage. The crew decided to turn back to Melbourne. Fuel had to be dumped to decrease the weight to a level acceptable for landing. How could it have come to this situation?

Data concerning wind direction, temperature, air pressure, runway length, and aircraft weight are entered into a computer by pilots independently of one another to ascertain numbers required for rotation and lift, flap setting, and engine power. In this case, time pressure resulted in only one pilot doing the calculations. Instead of entering a takeoff weight of 323 tons, he enters 232 tons. Switching these numbers means that this low (incorrect) weight results in the calculation of insufficient engine power and too low lift speed. The plane lacked the necessary velocity for a timely liftoff. There was no cross-check from the second pilot. Here too no one was injured. This was a blessing in disguise. Damages: 80 million US dollars.

Conclusion: Time pressure is highly dangerous. There is no reason to sacrifice safety to time constraints.

5.8   Crash Landing in Vienna

An Airbus A310 is on flight from Chania, Crete, to Hannover, Germany. The landing gear did not fully retract after takeoff; the pilots decided to continue the flight to Germany. The air drag caused by the partially extended landing gear resulted in fuel consumption higher than originally calculated.

Navigation computers base their calculations for fuel consumption on normal cruising altitude without considering technical difficulties. The estimated fuel consumption to the destination appeared for that reason to be sufficient. The actual consumption was, however, much higher and would require that the crew recalculate the amount.

The correct flight data plans for exceptional cases are to be found in the onboard manuals. During the flight, the fuel tanks went dry. The flight had to crash-land without fuel in Vienna. The flight could have been diverted to Budapest with the remaining fuel.

This is an example of a breakdown in teamwork. The captain pushed through his decision uncritically. The result was a total loss of the aircraft. His court hearing led to a prison sentence.

Lesson learned: Unusual circumstances require a reevaluation of all details of a process, to prevent overlooking unforeseen effects.

5.9   Error-Prevention Strategies

There is a long list of standard procedures in flight manuals which make safe flying possible. Before each flight, for example, every switch setting in the cockpit is checked over. Pilots must follow a flow pattern to insure that not one switch has been overlooked. For takeoff procedures, even hand movements, commands, and limits are listed in detail and are to be observed.

For this reason, checklists play an integral part in every phase of flight, from engine start-up to engine shutdown.

Mandatory procedures can be found in the so-called Quick Reference Handbook for everything from possible technical malfunctions to

emergencies involving fire onboard during flight or even to an emergency evacuation of passengers. Additionally for some situations, there are so-called memory items in which procedures must be memorized. Examples include starting an emergency descent, flying with complete loss of speed indicators or performing the precisely defined maneuvers to prevent a midair collision, just to name a few.

Despite an increase in flight-control automation, manual flying capabilities, or skills, are essential. We know that automation, the autopilot function, for example, can effectively assist and thereby relieve pilots in important phases of flight. This permits pilots to keep their heads clear for important decisions, especially during emergencies. Nonetheless, pilots must always be capable of manually flying the plane.

An analogy: A surgeon performing a high-tech operation must always be in a position to revert to conventional methods and to end a difficult operation without causing harm to the patient.

5.10   Aborted Takeoff Due to Engine Damage or Other Malfunctions

These decisions must be made within fractions of a second. This task is done by the captain only. There is no time for deliberation. The hand movements and procedures are performed automatically, in a drill-like fashion. These drills are trained in simulators regularly and at multiple times during the year.

An analogy: Drills are for the most part unknown in the field of medicine. In ambulances, for example, they could be quite helpful.

5.11   Loss of Engine Power During Takeoff or Climb

By figuring out performance data for takeoff, the captain and copilot define clear criteria by which takeoff could safely occur, even with engine loss.

During the cockpit briefing, relevant speeds are determined which allow for important decisions to be made explicitly well before takeoff: Up to what speed can the takeoff be aborted? Will we have to divert from the planned takeoff route in order to circumnavigate obstacles, and should we lose engine power and therefore our expected climb performance? Will we have to dump fuel? Where is our alternate airport in this particular situation?

A certain strategy is devised in these briefings which must be followed in case of an emergency. Time has been saved which would otherwise be needed for compulsory discussions. By coordinating these decisions, each pilot knows which strategy to follow in order to land the plane safely in an emergency.

Despite all the procedures going on in the cockpit, there is a strict separation between pilot flying (PF) and pilot not flying (PNF). The pilot flying is to concentrate solely on operating the aircraft, whether manually or with the help of the autopilot. The pilot nonflying oversees and observes the PF and takes over additional duties, such as completing the emergency checklist and maintaining communication with the cabin crew and with air traffic control via radio.

With this separation of duties, it is not always necessary for the captain to take over the role of pilot flying. At the same time, he must be able to assume the role at any time.

An analogy: A surgeon and assistant must perform their respective roles properly. The specialist functioning as trainer must be able to take over at any time.

5.12 Thunder Clouds En Route

Depending on the weather situation, severe thunderstorms may force a plane to divert from its planned route. Weather radar helps pilots to judge more precisely the weather situation and change route if necessary. Here too technology can aid immensely. Decisions have to, however, be made by the crew members themselves.

5.13 Aborted Approach

During an approach, various types of malfunctions can occur. There are clear limits which must be observed at all times. Here is an example for the final approach: speed +5/−0 knots, sink rate no more than 1000 ft/min, landing configurations no later than 300 m above ground, engine performance sufficiently set, and stabile approach. As a result of wind gusts, unexpected wind changes in direction or speed, these limits may be exceeded. In this case, the approach must be aborted. This is what is known as a "go-around." Should one of the two pilots doubt the safety of the situation, he must command a go-around. This command must be executed. The decision for a go-around under 300 m can also be made by the copilot. Should it later be determined that this decision was based on an error, there are no repercussions. It exemplified the safest course of action.

An analogy: A surgeon's assistant may and should express doubt; it is to be taken seriously.

5.14 Medical Emergencies Onboard

Medical emergencies unfortunately occur often. The average life span is increasing and for that reason also the number of elderly passengers on board. Circulatory collapses, heart attacks, and even deaths are situations for which we are dependent on professional, medical assistance. Often nurses, paramedics, and doctors are onboard who can offer this assistance.

Should there not be a doctor among the passengers, an alternative is to contact the Medical Assistance Center via satellite telephone. This 24-h service is staffed by doctors who offer medical support to airlines. This may result in a recommendation to divert to another airport en route, with full knowledge as to whether this airport is equipped with ample medical facilities or not. The next closest airport may not always have the equipment necessary for the particular cases on boards. In the future, it will even be possible to transmit important medical parameters via telemetry.

Pilots themselves are responsible for whether and to where a diversion occurs. The purely aeronautical criteria must first be evaluated by the crew: Is the airport able to handle this type of aircraft? Do their weather conditions permit a landing? Can the aircraft possibly take off from there again to bring hundreds of passengers to their original destination? The responsibility for these decisions remains always with the captain. He of course is supported by his team.

An analogy: Corrective decisions must be reviewed for their possibly unsolvable consequences before they can be implemented.

5.15 Loss of Pressure During Cruise

This circumstance requires quick decisions as this poses a direct danger to passengers' and crew members' lives. The so-called emergency descent must begin immediately. Within a few seconds, the cockpit must begin to use their 100 % oxygen supply in order to remain completely capable of acting. This scenario requires that both pilots work mostly independently of one another, even though the pilot flying continues to be monitored. Only after having reached a safe altitude can the cockpit crew decide at which airport to land under consideration of remaining fuel and medical attention for possibly injured passengers.

An analogy: One must be able treat an acute hemorrhage as an emergency while calmly trying to ascertain what is causing the bleeding and how to safely prevent it from reoccurring.

5.16 Risk of Bird Strike

This risk is especially present during takeoff and landing. Airports actively pursue bird determent. Still, a bird strike can cause problems such as a broken windshield or damaged engine. A spectacular example is of course the ditching of an A-320 in the Hudson River after takeoff from La Guardia Airport in New York. The situation escalated after two grey geese were ingested. Both engines became seriously damaged, resulting in a loss of thrust.

For this case – both engines shutting down at the same time – there is a procedure in the Quick Reference Handbook (QRH). That procedure would take several minutes to complete, a time period much too long for this emergency at the relatively low altitude of ca. 1000 m. In this case, the pilots had 2 min and 30 s until landing on the water. They were forced to perform quickly the most important procedures without a checklist.

Independent of one another, both pilots had to handle the situation meticulously. The captain glided the aircraft using only the emergency instruments and decided to perform a ditching. He briefly informed the cabin crew and passengers. The copilot activated those remaining technical systems which were needed and informed air traffic control about the impending ditching – certainly a brilliant performance by both pilots.

This example shows that under enormous pressure, decisions must be made. Even in this situation, both pilots functioned as a team. Their huge pool of experience allowed them to complete their respective tasks; they each knew what to do.

This fortunate outcome is the result of pilot competence, a professional sense of responsibility and effective cooperation within the crew, which saved not only the lives of all passengers but their own as well.

An analogy: Also in the medical field, ensuring recovery is a result of teamwork, not a result of individual ability.

5.17 Risk Reduction

The preparations for any flight are carried out by people of differing education levels, cultures, and abilities. For all involved, one dictum applies – safety first.

One decisive factor for flight safety is process discipline. This must be ensured even during times of stress.

A key to successful flying is an adequate amount of redundancy. The following serve as a net and double floor to achieve the highest possible level of safety:

- At least two of all systems and instruments are installed.
- All procedures are practiced in hands-on training in simulators.
- Training of critical flight phases takes place continually.
- Team conduct is strengthened through self-reflection.
- Training takes place in teams which strives to maximize error reduction.

An analogy: Redundancy as a way of ensuring (technical) safety is not well known in the field of medicine. The reason appears to be high costs. This must be seriously reconsidered.

In the development of flight systems, the human factor is also taken into account. It is crucial to combine technology and human being to prevent, on the one hand, pilots from becoming overburdened and, on the other hand, to ensure that the systems remain uncomplicated in their operation. The technology is not meant to replace the person but to support him in solving complex tasks.

If paper checklists describing procedures for every situation were used in the past, modern technology allows for planes to be equipped with warning computers in which checklists appear on the screen and which communicate interactively with the pilots.

Furthermore, aircraft manufacturers, aviation authorities, and airlines take part in investigations of aircraft irregularities and accidents. The results from these investigations help to improve safety.

All major airlines have a flight safety department headed by a captain. This department enjoys full trust and confidence by all pilots. All pilots are entreated to report flight occurrences either personally, via an ombudsman or even anonymously. Decisive is the joint responsibility. Share your experience.

How to Perform Risk Management

6

Walter Merkle

Abstract

There are principles in practical risk management to know; however, which technique for which problems to solve is crucial for success when dealing with risk management. This chapter will show these principles. Communication, checklists, CIRS, and simulator trainings are contents – and much more.

6.1 Introduction

In the first chapter of this textbook it was pointed out why doctors/medical staff need risk management which exceeds the management of medical risk of a given patient.

The so-called risk management deals with the inherent risk of a medical procedure – either in diagnostic or in therapy, because human behavior per se might cause mistakes.

In this chapter it will be shown which measures must be undertaken to reduce this imminent risk.

However, right at the beginning of this chapter it must be pointed out clearly that no complete solutions will be presented, ready to use, but rather tools to install and perform a good working risk management. Why? Whereas the principles of risk management are the same – both in a small and big facility or University hospital – the details are different. What is sufficient for a small low-volume hospital normally is insufficient for a University hospital.

A simple example might demonstrate this:

Appendectomy:
  Pathway: diagnosis – inpatient – recheck of correct diagnosis – information of the patient and formal consent of the operative procedure (appendectomy) – OR itself – postoperative care – discharging

Primary care hospital:
  Normally only a few people are working together, thus the doctor who sees the patient for the first time might be the same on the ward as well as in the OR to do the operation.

W. Merkle, MD
Riskmanager in Medicine Specialist in Urology,
Management Expert for Hospitals (VWA),
German Diagnostic Clinic – Helios Clinic,
Aukammallee 33, Wiesbaden D 65191, Germany
e-mail: Risikomanagement.Merkle@hotmail.de

© Springer-Verlag Berlin Heidelberg 2016
W. Merkle (ed.), *Risk Management in Medicine*, DOI 10.1007/978-3-662-47407-5_6

> Therefore this doctor knows everything about the patient and his special conditions, e.g. diabetes, coronary disease, etc., thus there is no lack of information between the patient's first step into the hospital till the operation. That means no risk of missing information.
>
> University hospital:
> The doctor in the ambulance who sees the patient first is not the same doctor on the ward. The surgeon most likely will not be the same colleague. And the postoperative care will be performed also by another doctor.
> It is obvious that important information might be lost during the patient's way from doctor to doctor with all possible consequences.

Patient care and patient safety
This is provided by
- ☐ Competence in the specific medical fields
- ☐ Competence in methods
- ☐ Competence in social affairs

The principal risks in the settings are

Quality in
- ☐ The medical discipline
- ☐ The structure
- ☐ The process itself

There isn't a hospital which can declare that every single point is absolutely correct.

Whoever believes this will soon be taught that this is definitely not the truth.

Even in the rare case this might be so for a short period – it remains mandatory to undertake any effort to stabilize this positive situation.

> Self satisfaction is the termination of any improvement! (Philipp Rosenthal).

6.2 Intersection Problems

Although it is a simple example, it is now clear that this book cannot describe all possibilities of medical errors and how to prevent them.

This book puts the seeds into the earth to let the plant of risk management grow.

The second example demonstrates clearly the problem due to intersection points in medical care. It is therefore mandatory to have a complete documentation on hand as soon as a patient will be transferred to another unit or to another doctor.

Information has to be up to date and complete.

All intersection points must be clearly defined to prevent loss of data. At all these points, a SOP (standard operation procedure) must commit to which information/results/documents have to be transferred from A to B.

Thus it is obvious that a University hospital needs SOPs much more than a small primary care hospital but the principles are the same.

The crucial processes of risk management are

6.3 Toolbox

Being totally aware of this principle, that especially in a hospital the human fact is all present and omnipotent, there is only one chance: to work as well as possible to reduce the amount of errors.

Avoidable errors must be consequently detected and deleted. But keep in mind that this is not a single process to be done but a permanent and continual process because the personnel changes regularly, thus renewing of training and rechecking the system are a permanent effort which will never stop.

Solid knowledge and sufficient training to improve abilities of the staff members is the aim. Interestingly, the more educated somebody is and the higher the cognitive capability, the higher is the risk awareness as a study at the Iowa State University showed (Cho and Orazem 2011).

Following strict guidelines is relatively common. Doing this is to be valued only as minor management quality which leads to minor quality results, because sticking to guidelines would suspend great potential of success.

Therefore the first claim is that the hospital's administration should be open for suggestions from their staff which thereafter should be put into action in cooperation between staff and administration. To accept this, it is not necessary for the administration to understand all details but to trust the capability of the staff members to nominate their best experts.

Sometimes coaching (see Chap. 8) can support this behavior.

Project groups therefore are good and successful tools to solve even complex and difficult problems with many interfaces (=a lot of people involved).

To make such groups even quicker, it is helpful if the leader is experienced in moderation training.

Again this example points out clearly that the personal capability of the staff members is the key to success. Investment in training is reimbursed.

Communication skills in both directions: leader$<->$staff must work together whenever and wherever without bureaucratic obstacles (see CRM, Chap. 14).

Sure, in a big company it is impossible that everybody has free access to the higher management, but in smaller companies the management should know almost everybody.

The critical point of large organizations is the transparency between high and low, between chief of department and trainee, nurses and doctors, etc. Everybody must be aware of transparency to avoid missing information which might be crucial for patient's health. Good communication needs self-discipline, especially when using email ("putting a long list into "cc"): distribute important things, document information of minor importance for further questioning, which will not be distributed routinely. Thus, important information will not be overlooked in the daily machine-gun shooting of emails.

Example:
Although it is the duty of the administration to close a ward it should be absolutely possible that even a low-ranking staff member might phone the administration office directly in case of emergency when, e.g., the hot heating tube is lacking. Thus immediate and direct information can reduce risk and harm for patients by contact with hot water.

The bureaucratic way of information in such a case would cost too much time until the administration would have a chance to react, evacuate the patients, and close the ward for repair.

6.3.1 Risk Management Strategies

The simplest method of risk strategy is to buy insurance. This will reduce the financial cost of mistakes; however, being insured might also cause the opposite – not being sure but unsure – as the risk awareness can become minor because of relying on the insurance policy.

Furthermore, the patient's injury cannot be valued by money; money cannot bring back health. And the damage of a hospital's image might be much greater than loss of money.

Thus insurance reduces money-like risk but cannot prevent a hospital from bankruptcy.

Therefore reduction of failure costs is the aim which will reduce the insurance premium (Chap. 18).

To achieve this, the probability of failures must be reduced by learning, e.g., when reading this textbook.

Learning means to send staff members to training (although they will be out of work for a certain period). Thus this costs money.

To say it clearly, risk management does cost investment of money, but without investing money and training staff, risk management will fail (Chambers 2010).

As Morita pointed out, "Healthcare institutions are known to be risky environments that still lay behind other industries in the development and application of risk management tools. … Risk awareness is calibrated to the true risk levels of the institutions (risk awareness and safety culture)" (Morita et al. 2011).

Consequently hospitals must build up awareness that they cover significant risks which are not fate but can be reduced by sufficient methods.

The ECRI Institute (www.ecri.org) in 2011 has published a list how a working risk management system should be established.

Mandatory for a Risk Management System

☐ Risk management system must have open access for all staff members (not exclusively for the administration).

☐ RM program must be visible for the staff.

☐ The complete staff must be trained in RM programs (training is obliged).

☐ Complete results must be open and available.

☐ List of all RM activities.

☐ Support of RM program's use.

Further conditions are motivation of staff, support and engagement of the hospitals' administration, continuous training, and a consequent culture of confidence; it is obvious to provide sufficient resources (personal and financial).

There are typical errors due to the structure of a hospital. Additionally, to err is human, thus doctors' behavior has to anticipate these points and must steer against them. Risk management protects both patients and doctors.

Example:

Long distance for patient's transport – reduced capacity of elevators; poor print quality of lab report:

Too long time for transport between ward and OR, e.g., or intensive care unit might urge the transport team to be accompanied by a doctor for safety reasons – this costs money.

Poor readable lab result can cause overlooking of important results causing improper therapy which can lead to the patient's harm (I had such a case as expert for the court).

6.3.2 Risk Analysis

As soon as all members of the RM process agree and resources are available, the very beginning is a complete analysis of all processes and working fields. No taboo is allowed.

Afterward because the tsunami of information can hardly be handled, 5–10 major problems are addressed which are intuitively found without a certain analysis because they are obvious for insiders.

After the first experiences, a systemic analysis of the complete hospital has to follow.

But where to begin? A peer review might help to identify the most important risk zones (Chap. 13).

A simple but effective marker of the hospital's risk areas can be found in the complaints which patients – mostly anonymously – post to the administration. Following them is relatively simple to reduce the risk situation. A further advantage of this simple act is the patient's impression: They reacted to my complaint and improved the process.

This improves satisfaction of patients and image of the hospital. And – not to underestimate – staff members' satisfaction will improve as well as their motivation.

Cydulka et al. (2011) could demonstrate in 34 emergency units in 8 US states that just by this simple method significant problems could be removed prior to patients' injury.

Errors must be visible to enable a prospective management to avoid them.

This procedure is mandatory because avoidable errors are principally counted as malpractice, thus legal proceedings will be lost and insurance companies might refuse to pay. Thus the legal consequences must be paid by the hospital itself even if the sum might be high.

There are not only the costs of regulation and patient injury but also the costs of longer hospital stay due to error-caused injury which will not lead to refunding by the patient or his insurance company. Therefore the hospital's EBIT will decrease.

Not installing risk management increases the risk of the hospital's survival at the market

When working with these processes, attention must be paid to performing systems and processes to originate more tolerance to possible errors before they might injure a patient and cost the hospital's money.

This prospective work is more or less the entire heart zone. How to perform this can be found in the chapter on FMEA (Chap. 11).

Checklists and control points must be established, e.g., where a four-eyes principle is mandatory, for example, when transferring a patient from the OR to the ICU or ICU to routine ward. A form can support this. Then the transfer is robust against errors of incomplete information from one point of care to another.

Therefore it reduces costs and effort when these checkpoints are planned right at the beginning of establishing a pathway.

6.3.3   Documentation Is Mandatory

Documentation is mandatory as follows:

☐ Four-eyes principle for all operations with bilateral organs
☐ Check of patient's name when entering the OR area by actively asking the patient for his/her name
☐ Repeat all orders which contain a sum or dosage of drug therapy
☐ Written documentation of all orders

These rules of documentation are enforced by law and courts. Additionally the ISO 9001:200

and ISO 15,224 respectively point this out absolutely clearly.

Part of this documentation process is a regular check of documentation quality. For this a SOP (standard operation process) has to be established (Chap. 21).

6.3.4   Practical Work

After the more intuitive kick-off meeting in risk management, a systematic and frankly open analysis of the current status has to be performed.

Because of the overwhelming amount of things to do at the beginning, it is wise to start with Pareto's diagram, which can show the most frequent errors which must be analyzed and solved first.

It is well known that only 5–10 frequent errors are responsible for approximately 80 % of total errors.

Thus the primary workload is limited and will lead to positive results very soon.

6.3.5   How to Analyze Errors?

☐ Repeated (same) errors in the complete hospital (most likely a structural problem!)
☐ Most expensive errors (largest amount of money, largest loss of economic reputation)
☐ Departments with the most complaints
☐ Repeated and most common complaints
☐ Staff member interview for most important problems
☐ Department with the lowest ROI
☐ CIRS report/results
☐ Importance of errors (first, human being and/or most important process for the hospital)
☐ Results of FMEA

6.3.6   Clinical Pathways

The aim of the zero-failure strategy can be reached when clinical pathways are analyzed in project groups and thereafter are optimized or newly set up adopting the individual situation of the hospital.

The principle of the DMAIC cycle (Chap. 1) has proven successful as soon as the problems are *committed* through the risk analysis. The typical pathway of all doings and all participants of a given process are described.

When doing this it is absolutely mandatory not to overlook simple actions which seem to be a matter of course, because it can happen that this simple action can recover the point at which the process does not go smoothly.

One typical example of such a simple but important process that everybody in a hospital knows is the ordering of patients to be brought to the OR. It can cost more time to change patients on the table when the simple transportation of the next scheduled patient takes too long.

But why doesn't anyone change this? Solving this transportation problem from status quo to "just in time" is qualified to be the first step of training when establishing risk management.

Someone might think this transportation problem is not really worth engaging in, but let's not forget in case of an urgent operation every minute counts. Furthermore, overtime work costs additional money which reduces in the last consequence the hospital's return.

And also not to forget, the whispering of patients concerning such a transportation chaos.

Next, because human factors are the most important source of errors, it is wise to start there with training staff and solve obvious problems (Chap. 4).

Because dealing with human error is very complex, it is helpful and makes things much easier if we look abroad where others successfully have solved human-factor problems – and how they did it (Chap. 5).

The most experienced human factor solutions are found in the airline business.

Watching pilots' work in their cockpit leads to interesting observations:

Communication and hierarchy are both most important terms which are directly linked to errors and fatal consequences including total loss. Details can be found in the "air business" chapters.

That the load of examples and experience from the air business is clever might show this:

In the *Journal of Urology* which normally reports about medical contexts, there was an interesting article in 2011 by Erickson and Boulanger:

> John Nance, a pilot and member of the American National Patient Safety Foundation, reported how his request to a young pilot trainee to tell him everything which might cause fear was paid back by saving their lives.
>
> During the plane's ascent, the control tower ordered flight level 15. The pilot (J. Nance) understood flight level 17. The trainee called the pilot's attention to the wrong flight level and thus avoided a possible accident. Through the correction to the correct flight level, a jumbo jet flying above them was not hurt. If the trainee would have been too shy to call the experienced pilot's attention to the situation, over 300 people would have died!

The consequence drawn in this article was learning from the pilots!

Flat hierarchy was the key to safe lives!

Additionally, more or less the reported behavior is part of the so-called CRM – crew resource management. In Chap. 14 an important report to CRM can be found.

Two points I do want to pick from this chapter to show the importance of CRM. First, it is mandatory that everybody clearly understands that he is member of a team and that he does make mistakes.

In a team there are different duties to do, thus no team member is unnecessary.

For example, although the cleaning service personnel is found at the bottom of a hospital's hierarchy, these people are equally important because without cleaning the wastepaper basket it would not be long until the administration would drown in paper masses.

The "normal" human behavior of looking down on lower-ranking people is not wise and does not lead to the goal of running any business smoothly and successfully. Over time only a team is able to solve problems and work successfully.

Therefore Burke was correct when he wrote, " how to turn a team of experts into an expert medical team: guidance from aviation and military communities" (Burke et al. 2004).

Second, higher-ranking team members have to listen to lower-ranking team members in case the lower-ranking members say they have concerns.

This is not insubordination but expression of serious concerns – eventually pointing to the most important and crucial process to be bewared to fail.

Imagine – a service staff member would not tell the chief surgeon that the patient on the table is Mr. Smith and not Mr. Miller. The day before, the service staff member had spoken to the patient himself, thus knowing who he is. The chief surgeon might not have seen the patient prior to the operation for which he was selected due to his special expertise but not because the patient is one of his own clients. Thus uncovering the name error would prevent doing the wrong operation to the wrong patient. (Therefore during TTO identification of the patient is mandatory)

This example might look as if it is artificially constructed. Well, the society of surgeons has adopted those identification problems and put the question for the patient's name onto the preoperative checklist!

I sometimes find that a new patient comes into my office when the next patient is called although another patient with a different name was called! How can this be explained?

Temporary lack of attention can be presumed although people find nothing more important than their own name. The second explanation can be found in stress.

Both conditions will be explained in another part in the textbook.

6.3.7   Checklists

Checklists definitely improve patient safety.

This was shown clearly in a study at Harvard University with 7700 patients. Half of them were examined prior to establishing checklists, half of them thereafter. The average complication ratio decreased when using checklists from 11 to 7 %, and the death rate decreased from 1.5 to 0.8 %. This is a 40 % reduction (Haynes et al. 2009)!

However, checklists are not a universal cure for everything. They are not equally usable for each hospital. Also in this condition there are differences between a small local hospital and a hospital built for maximum care (Chap. 1).

Checklists are made to be remembered, enable complete work, thus not overlooking essentials. But each individual hospital has to form its own checklist.

And this individual checklist must be filled with life. Adaption by time is desired and should correspond to the DMAIC cycle.

Checklists also assist when the situation is hectic or when work (emergency room!) must be done at unusual times or during weekends when there is not the routine team in charge but special conditions are present. It is known that the amount of risks depend on the working hour. Sleep deprivation leads to errors.

Drivers know that; why not doctors of medicine?

In case an operation is necessary due to an emergency condition, the mentioned techniques help to reduce the imminent risk of such a special condition – meaning checklist, TTO, OTAS, CRM, etc. See the specific chapters.

However, checklists are able to detect errors *in* minor quality organizations and processes. There they can help to avoid or solve them. But human-caused errors are not detectable by checklists. To reduce or prevent this kind of error interaction between human beings, meaning by team interaction, their optimized handling of a problem is essential. This is CRM (see Chap. 14).

6.3.8   The Problems of Formal Consent

A very important point inside any checklist is the so-called formal consent.

It permits a doctor to perform all kinds of treatment, even an operation. Especially in

Germany, this formal consent is crucial because an operation is legally an injury of the patient's body, thus punishable. For the specific German details see the German version of this textbook, published in February 2014 with Springer, Heidelberg.

For the specific legal version for USA and Europe, see Chaps. 16 and 17.

6.3.9 CIRS

Critical incident reporting system – at present this is the most commonly performed act of risk management in medicine. For details see Chap. 9.

However, CIRS tells us that something almost went wrong. Thus, CIRS reports about errors or almost errors.

In case the CIRS report would be the only consequence of such a faulty situation it would have cost money and would be worthless.

CIRS will be a useful tool in risk management only if consequences in daily practice will be drawn, especially in case the near mistake is of systematic value.

In case consequences were drawn and a process would have been changed it remains also important to re-evaluate whether the changes were successful or might have brought new errors.

Therefore it is absolutely mandatory to combine CIRS with other techniques of risk management such as DMAIC cycle, FMEA, FORDEC, and RADAR.

These techniques are commonly and successfully used even in sensitive areas such as airlines, space technology, chemistry and the nuclear field, etc..

For details see the specific chapters. For a glance,

☐ FMEA: Failure mode and effect analysis: this means think in advance which problems might occur when doing something. The consequences are estimated and tools were developed to reduce the risk or even prevent error and negative consequences of the specific process. To achieve this best an interdisciplinary team is built where many different insights can be combined to have an almost complete overview thereafter. This prevents lacks in a process.

☐ RADAR: Result-Approach-Deployment-Assessment-Review: this is comparable to FMEA and also a scheme how a process can run. First the error is analyzed, e.g., which was detected by CIRS, then an appropriate way of solution is fixed. Thereafter virtually (!) the solution is evaluated by a project team, the results are evaluated again, and then a positively proven process will be activated to eliminate the former error in reality.

☐ FORDEC: Facts-Option-Risks-Decision-Execution-Check: FORDEC is also an established method of x-ray procedures, processes, errors, etc.. Compared to RADAR, FORDEC has the advantage to prethink risks and potential errors - FORDEC is more or less a combination of RADAR, FMEA, and DMAIC.

☐ DMAIC: This is the quality management cycle. It is organized by strictly using the cycle steps to think over a process or error and look for improvement.

Thus DMAIC is the best of all the mentioned techniques.

Very important to mention is that everything, really everything without any exception is laid on the table. This also includes

☐ Out-of-date equipment
☐ Not enough staff members
☐ Missed training of staff
☐ Unacceptable buildings
☐ *Unproved* modernization ("flying on untested wings")
☐ Shortage of equipment due to saving or lacking of money

Sometimes even when carefully following these error-mode techniques it might be impossible to detect the cause. Then a peer review process might be of value and helpful.

6.3.10 Peer Review

Why in such a situation might PR be further helpful? The most decisive advantage of PR is the evaluation of one's own hospital through an outside expert (Chap. 13).

Normally the PR process is organized as follows: The leading physicians of the hospital invite colleagues from another hospital to check their procedures.

Because these colleagues are experienced in the processes they should observe it is not necessary to explain details – this is the crucial – and important! – difference when compared with QM teams which only look for formalistic protocols but mostly do not understand anything from the things they have to review.

The peer review team is not blind to the organization they have to review, because they have an outside view and insight. By this PR method normally even hidden errors are detected and can be changed thereafter.

PR is a specific procedure which needs much sensitivity of all PR team members to be honest and avoiding sneering. Furthermore the results must be absolutely confidential because the reviewed hospital is being exposed in areas which are normally not public.

However, without this very deep insight PR would not work.

It is ideal when both involved hospital teams invite each other. Thus confidence would build up even better. And the learning effect doubles.

6.3.11 Communication

The word "communication" is a key term in risk management.

Communication is crucial between doctors and administration. Only in the case of working together confidentially will it be possible to reduce the imminent risk of running a hospital and treating patients. When the communication is open and frank, a quadruple multiwin situation is created – for patients, doctors, staff members, and the administration (and owners).

More or less this multiwin situation is the aim of this textbook on risk management in hospitals.

6.3.12 Simulator Training

The permanent links to the airline business leads to the obvious question: why is there almost no simulator training in medicine?

The answer is simple – the common operation techniques can hardly be simulated with a machine; they open the belly, the thorax, or replace a hip, etc..

The modern techniques using minimally invasive equipment can be trained with a simulator. This contains, e.g., *transurethral* procedures of the prostate, laparoscopic operations, and even more robotic techniques (daVinci roboter).

This is part of virtual learning which meanwhile is widespread. Although it is rather expensive, the effort is paid back (Wenderlein 2012). The unavoidable learning curve thus can be reduced which saves money and increases safety of patients. Dummy training is free of risk and helps training step by step which improves the manual capability of the surgeon.

But not to forget – in a simulator nobody can reach his holiday hotel; nobody can cure a patient there. The test of capability will take place with a real patient in the last consequence.

Simulator training must not be followed by the trainee's opinion that he is perfect and able to do a real-life procedure. Simulator training is just for increased speed for the learning curve.

However, brilliant actions such as Captain Sullenberger's landing on the Hudson River are prepared by multiple simulator trainings. Thus unconscious behavior is trained which can be recalled without too much conscious thinking and directly put into active action. Only the intellectual thinking processes must be done, and this can be performed even under stress.

This, together with CRM, is the "mystery" behind success.

The next problem with simulator training is "flying on untested wings" because one might have the opinion of being perfect. Especially in medicine this is a real problem. It can happen that a new procedure is brought to almost routine without testing sufficiently.

The only good news is that most of these procedures disappear within a short period, eventually due to complications. The test of time has failed.

Therefore, in case a new procedure is brought to clinical use it must be accompanied by serious quality control to detect complications, etc. as soon as possible. Furthermore, patients have to be informed that this is a new, not completely proven technique they should undergo. The patient should be asked to report all – even minor – events after such new operation techniques.

Conclusion

Every single error is one error too many.

Therefore all efforts must be undertaken to avoid it. This is only possible when everyone is ready to accept to report failures even if they are by themselves.

Kaizen – thank you that I was permitted to learn from your mistakes.

A good established life risk management system is targeted to reach this aim.

The risk analysis must be performed at the very beginning. Thereafter the process can start.

Important is

☐ Open communication with all staff members and all involved partners as well as the administration
☐ Avoiding top-down procedures but commonly acting together
☐ Avoiding hierarchy
☐ Learning capability – everybody from everybody
☐ Introduction of a complaint management
☐ Introduction of a proposal system by staff members
☐ Accepting personal responsibility

All staff members of a hospital sit in the same boot.

Acting – not reacting – to avoid failures is necessary.

By the way, a well-functioning risk management system can be a good marking aspect. Some big hospital groups use this aspect.

And a glance into literature can be helpful.

In urology the open discussion of errors and which consequences can be drawn is standard. Meanwhile, several textbooks were written dealing with this; unfortunately all are published in German (Steffens and Langen 2002, 2005; Anheuser and Steffens 2012). And at scientific congresses the theme is regularly present. Meanwhile the EAU had developed a guideline. The first is written for Iatrogenic Trauma (Summerton et al. 2012).

These activities are exemplary. Errors are reported, experts draw conclusions, and everybody can learn from it thereafter.

Thus even an error has a good aspect – somehow.

Literature

Chambers DW (2010) Risk management. J AM Coll Dent 77:35–45

Cydulka RK, Tamayo-Sarver J, Gage A, Bagnoli D (2011) Association of patient satisfaction with complaints and risk management among emergency physicians. J Emerg Med 41:405–11

Eur Urol (2012) 82:628–639

Haynes AB, Weiser TG, Berry WR, Lipsitz SR, Breizat A-HS, Dellinger EP, Herbosa T, Joseph S, Kibatala PL, Lapitan MCM, Merry AF, Moorthy K, Reznick RK, Taylor B, Gawande AA, for the Safe Surgery Saves Lives Study Group (2009) A Surgical Safety Checklist to Reduce Morbidity and Mortality in a Global Population. N Engl J Med 360:491–499

MBZ 12/24. August 2012

Morita PP et al (2011) Situation awareness and risk management understanding the notification issues. Stud Health Technol Inform 164:372–76

Cho and Orazem (2011) Working paper No. 11016, Aug. 2011

Patient safety: above and beyond the checklist (2011) J Urol 185:1177–1178

Qual Saf Health Care (2004) Suppl 13:196

Steffens J, Langen P-H (Hrsg) (2012) Komplikationen in der Urologie, Steinkopff, Darmstadt 2002; Komplikationen in der Urologie 2, Steinkopff, Darmstadt 2005; P. Anheuser, J. Steffens (Hrsg.): Risiken und Komplikationen in der Urologie. Thieme, Stuttgart

Hospital Risk Management and the U.S. Legal System: An Introduction to U.S. Medical Malpractice Tort Law

7

C.J. Stimson

Abstract

In the US hospital setting, risk management focuses on mitigating hospital exposure to loss from legal liability, including medical malpractice tort law claims. This chapter provides perspective on three critical components of the US medical malpractice tort law: process, substance, and justification. Framed in this way, the discussion that follows illuminates both the practice and the policy that forms the foundation of US medical malpractice tort law.

7.1 Introduction

Risk management focuses on mitigating an enterprise's exposure to loss. In the hospital setting, one of the primary loss exposures is from legal liability. Legal liability can flow from multiple legal sources, including common law, statutory law, and administrative law. In this chapter, we will review a specific subset of the US common law of torts: medical malpractice law. Specifically, we will investigate the process, substance, and justification of US medical malpractice tort law.

C.J. Stimson, MD, JD
Department of Urologic Surgery, Vanderbilt University Medical Center, Nashville, TN, USA
e-mail: cj.stimson@vanderbilt.edu

7.2 Medical Malpractice Tort Law: Defined

In the US, patients who are injured as a result of negligent medical care can pursue legal remedy under the common law of torts (Stimson et al. 2010). The common law is a set of rules derived from judicial precedent, rather than rules issued by legislative bodies or administrative agencies, and includes tort law as a specific subset of common law focusing on civil injuries (Black 1999). Specifically, tort law determines whether an individual whose actions harm another should be required to pay compensation for the harm done (Franklin and Rabin 2006). In medical malpractice law, the query focuses on whether an injured patient is legally entitled to monetary compensation from the physician alleged to have harmed the patient.

© Springer-Verlag Berlin Heidelberg 2016
W. Merkle (ed.), *Risk Management in Medicine*, DOI 10.1007/978-3-662-47407-5_7

7.3   Medical Malpractice Tort Law: Process

Legal claims of medical malpractice are initiated through the US judicial system. Although there are extrajudicial means of pursuing relief for civil injuries, this section will highlight the process for pursuing legal remedy through US courts. The parties to this procedure include those claiming the injury (i.e., plaintiffs), those alleged to have perpetrated the injury (i.e., tortfeasors or defendants), the attorneys for these parties, the judge, and potentially a jury. This chapter will use the plaintiff and defendant nomenclature, although in medical malpractice tort law, this typically refers to the patient and physician, respectively.

To initiate a medical malpractice claim, the injured patient must file a complaint describing both the facts and the legal justification for a court-enforced remedy. The complaint is presented to the court and the healthcare provider, serving as notice to the provider that they are the target of a civil legal action. The provider will then be given a specific period of time to respond to the complaint (Franklin and Rabin 2006).

The defendant has several options once notified of the complaint, including moving to dismiss the claim based on insufficient legal grounds or refuting the facts presented in the complaint. Challenging the legal theory behind a plaintiff's complaint is a "demurrer," wherein the defendant argues that regardless of the veracity of the alleged facts, there is no legal cause of action to support the plaintiff's claims (The pleading and demurrer problems re-examined – new proposals in New York 1960). If the judge finds the defendant's demurrer persuasive, then the plaintiff's case will be dismissed. However, if the judge denies the demurrer, then the plaintiff's legal cause of action will stand, and the defendant must contest the facts of the complaint or accept them and be a subject to liability (Franklin and Rabin 2006). To challenge the facts in the complaint, as opposed to the law, the defendant files a pleading referred to as the "answer," and as a fact dispute, this is under the purview of a jury rather than a judge.

At this point, it is useful to distinguish between disputes over law and disputes over facts and how these disputes are treated differently by medical malpractice tort law. Generally, the US common law grants judges the authority to resolve disputes over the law while leaving disputes over facts to a jury (Havighurst et al. 1998). It would be reasonable and generally correct to infer from this rule that jury trials are therefore required when a plaintiff's complaint and a defendant's answer raise a question of fact. A notable exception is with a motion for summary judgment.

A defendant's motion for summary judgment argues that a judge should dismiss a medical malpractice tort claim without a jury trial because there is no genuine dispute over the facts (Brunet 1988). To succeed in this motion, the defendant must provide evidence demonstrating that there are no material issues of fact for a jury to resolve (*McGuckin v. Smith* 1992). If the moving party fails to provide convincing evidence, then the motion fails. If, however, the judge determines that the defendant has presented sufficient evidence to support summary judgment, then the plaintiff now carries the evidentiary burden of proving that there is a triable issue of fact. A plaintiff that is unable to meet this evidentiary burden will have their complaint dismissed on the grounds that a jury trial is unnecessary (Franklin and Rabin 2006).

To illustrate the concept of summary judgment, consider the case of *Alvarez v. Prospect Hospital et al.* (1986). During an evaluation for abdominal pain, the plaintiff was diagnosed by a radiologist with "cecal neoplasm" based on radiographic findings. The radiologist's final interpretation was submitted to the patient's attending physician who discharged her from the hospital with a diagnosis of gastroenteritis but without any mention of the radiologist's cancer finding. The patient ultimately underwent surgical treatment for her colon cancer, but this was delayed, and the patient filed a complaint under medical malpractice tort law against the attending physician and radiologist.

During the course of the litigation, the radiologist filed a motion for summary judgment, arguing that there was no triable issue of fact because he had accurately interpreted the radiographic findings and relayed this data to the patient's attending physician. On appeal, the court agreed with the radiologist, holding that there was no factual dispute rebutting the radiologist's claim that he "properly and timely diagnosed the plaintiff's condition and did not depart from the accepted standard of care in the medical community." Therefore, the court granted the radiologist's motion for summary judgment and dismissed the complaint against him. Notably, it was the plaintiff's reliance on the accuracy of the radiologist's report in her claim against her attending physician that proved fatal to her affidavit opposing the radiologist's motion for summary judgment.

Once the judge concurs that the plaintiff has a legal cause of action and there is a genuine issue of fact, the case then proceeds to a jury trial. The jury trial for a medical malpractice tort case is similar to other trials under tort law, except for the role of expert medical witnesses that will be discussed later. The plaintiff carries the burden of proving to the jury that the facts of the case satisfy the legal requirements for liability. To satisfy this burden, the plaintiff must present evidence supporting her own theory of events while also discrediting the evidence proffered by the defendant. The burden of proof can vary from state to state, including "more likely than not" or "a preponderance of the evidence." Once both parties have finished presenting their evidence, they proceed with closing arguments to persuade the jury that the circumstances favor either the plaintiff or defendant. Finally, before the jury proceeds to deliberation to consider a verdict, the judge instructs the jury about the legal rules they need to apply to their interpretation of the facts (Franklin and Rabin 2006).

It is important to note that common law judges have significant authority to alter the outcome of a jury trial. Prior to jury deliberation, the judge can dismiss the case or rule in favor of the plaintiff if the presented evidence is such that a jury can only reach one conclusion. This is referred to as a "directed verdict" or "judgment as a matter of law" and is done in response to a motion by either the plaintiff or defendant (*Fay v. Grand*

Strand Regional Medical Center, LLC 2015). Following the jury's verdict, a judge can vacate the verdict or order a new trial if all of the evidence overwhelmingly indicates that no contrary verdict could ever stand or if the judge believes the jury was influenced by a factor other than the facts presented, respectively (*Pedrick v. Peoria and Eastern RR Co* 1967; *York v. Rush-Presbyterian-St. Luke's* 2006). In both instances, the judge wields considerable authority to supplant the role of the jury.

Once a jury verdict rules in favor of the plaintiff, the next step is determining the damages the plaintiff is entitled to. Calculated as a lump-sum monetary payment, the total damage award is the summation of compensatory and punitive damages. Compensatory damages attempt to restore a plaintiff to their condition prior to the injury, while punitive damages are awarded as punishment and deterrence against certain conduct (Black 1999).

Compensatory damages can be further divided into pecuniary and nonpecuniary damages (*Fein v. Permanente Medical Group* 1985). Pecuniary damages are measureable losses, both past and future, and typically include medical expenses and lost earnings (*Greer v. Advantage Health* 2014). Nonpecuniary damages are for nonmeasurable losses and are often described as damages for "pain and suffering" (Chang et al. 2014). Although beyond the scope of this chapter, it is important to note that tort reform efforts in the US often focus on placing limits on certain types of damages.

Punitive damages are available upon findings of "actual malice" by the defendant and are only available as an adjunct to compensatory damages. Actual malice is defined as either: (1) conduct characterized by hatred, ill will, or revenge or (2) a conscious disregard for the rights and safety of other persons (*Preston v. Murty* 1987). To illustrate, consider the facts of *Moskovitz v. Mt. Sinai Medical Center*. At trial, the jury found that the physician provided negligent medical care and included punitive damages because the physician destroyed medical records to conceal evidence of the negligence. The defendant appealed the punitive component of the damage award, arguing that destroying medical records did not result in any harm to the plaintiff. The appellate court disagreed, holding the following:

> An intentional alteration, falsification or destruction of medical records by a doctor, to avoid liability for his or her medical negligence, is sufficient to show actual malice, and punitive damages may be awarded whether or not the act of altering, falsifying or destroying records directly causes compensable harm. (Moskovitz v. Mt. Sinai Med. Ctr 1994)

Finally, the amount of damages awarded is a fact question first committed to the discretion of the jury and next to the discretion of the judge if there is a motion for a new trial. Defendants who appeal damage awards as being excessive must overcome significant deference by appellate courts to awards issued at the trial court level. The only damage awards vacated by an appellate court are those that are so high that it "shocks the conscience and gives rise to the presumption that [the award] was the result of passion or prejudice on the part of the jurors" (*Seffert v. Los Angeles Transit Lines* 1961; *Hodgson v. Bigelow* 1939).

The medical malpractice tort law process is nuanced and deliberate. The distinctive approach to questions of law and fact is a key feature. In the following section, the substance of the legal questions and the framing of the factual debate will be discussed in more detail.

7.4 Medical Malpractice Tort Law: Substance

The dispositive legal question in medical malpractice tort is whether the healthcare provider was negligent in the performance of a professional act (*Hodgson v. Bigelow* 1939). The negligence analysis requires a two-part inquiry. The plaintiff must demonstrate that: (1) the healthcare provider owed a duty to the patient and (2) the duty was breached (Stimson et al. 2010; Studdert et al. 2004). Once negligence has been established, the plaintiff must prove that the defendant's negligence was the cause of an injury (*Hightower-Warren v. Silk* 1997). In the paragraphs that follow, these elements will be further explored.

7.4.1 Duty

The existence of healthcare provider's duty to a patient is predicated on the physician-patient relationship (*Kelley v. Middle Tenn.* Emergency Physicians 2004; *Church v. Perales* 2000; *Darby v. Union Planters National Bank of Memphis* 1969), transforming the initial negligence analysis into a question about whether a physician-patient relationship exists. To demonstrate this relationship, the plaintiff must prove that they – expressly or impliedly – sought professional assistance from the physician and that the physician – expressly or impliedly – agreed to treat the patient (*Jennings v. Case* 1999). This relationship does not require that the patient and physician meet in person or that a formal contractual agreement be arranged (*Lownsbury v. VanBuren* 2002) and includes attending physicians supervising resident trainees at teaching hospitals (*Mozingo v. Pitt County Memorial Hosp and Inc* 1992; *Maxwell v. Cole* 1984; *McCullough v. Hutzel Hospital* 1979). In other words, a patient-physician relationship exists when there is evidence indicating that the physician is acting in the patient's best interest (*Lownsbury v. VanBuren* 2002).

7.4.2 Breach

The next step in the negligence analysis is to determine whether a physician breached their legal duty to provide medical care for the plaintiff. To succeed in this analysis, the plaintiff must both establish the standard of care relevant to the medical circumstances of the case and present evidence that the physician failed to meet this standard (*Komlodi v. Picciano* 2014). The standard of care inquiry often serves as the dispositive issue in medical malpractice tort law cases, and the nuances of defining this standard merit further discussion.

7.4.2.1 Standard of Care: Definition and Justification

The standard of care inquiry in medical malpractice cases is distinct from that seen in other tort litigations. Unlike other tort cases where customary practice *informs but does not define* the standard of care, the standard of care in medical malpractice tort *is defined by* professional medical custom (Regan 1956). This heightened professional standard requires that medical experts provide testimony to inform the questions of fact and law before the court. Interestingly, this deference to the medical profession is both a shield and a sword. While allowing professional custom to define the legal standard protects medical decision-making from the scrutiny of the laity, it can also expose defendants to more scrupulous peer review.

The unique approach to the standard of care analysis in medical malpractice tort law is a deviation from the typical judicial treatment of allegedly tortious conduct and therefore demands legal justification. Toward this end, there is a well-established jurisprudence supporting the medical profession's unique self-regulatory legal status. The most persuasive line of reasoning argues that fact finders, including both judges and jury members, lack the specialized training and knowledge required to properly determine what reasonable and prudent actions a similarly situated physician would take (McCoid 1958). Further reasoning posits that expropriating the professional self-regulation of the legal standard of care to the nonmedical community could negatively impact patient care quality (McCoid 1958). Stated otherwise, the traditional tort standard of care analysis could result in low-quality medical care by exposing medical judgments to uninformed, ex post oversight rather than professional standards.

7.4.2.2 Standard of Care: Expert Witnesses' Testimony

The previous discussion highlights the need for expert witness testimony in defining the standard of care; however, the practical question regarding what testimony is admissible as evidence in medical malpractice tort cases remains. Answering this question requires an analysis of the jurisprudence underlying the admissibility of expert medical testimony. The US Supreme Court decision in *Daubert v. Merrill Dow Pharmaceutical Company* (1993)

and its subsequent progeny represent the most relevant contemporary line of case law on the topic.

Prior to the *Daubert* decision, the "general acceptance" test from *Frye v. United States* (1923) was the established standard for the admissibility of expert scientific evidence in medical malpractice litigation. The *Frye* ruling, from the court of appeals for the District of Columbia, held that a "scientific principle" is allowable as evidence before a finder of fact if the principle is "sufficiently established to have gained general acceptance in the particular field in which it belongs" (*Frye v. United States* 1923). This deferential standard allowed the "particular field" to guide the admissibility of expert testimony rather than judges.

The 1993 US Supreme Court decision in *Daubert* redirected 70 years of common law jurisprudence following *Frye* (*Daubert v. Merrell Dow Pharmaceuticals, Inc* 1993). Finding that the Federal Rules of Evidence, passed by the US Congress in 1975, superseded the common law from *Frye*, the justices weaved a new standard incorporating elements both from *Frye* and the statutory rules of evidence. The standard included four elements built on the idea that falsifiability is the hallmark of scientific enterprise: (1) the theory or technique can be and has been tested; (2) the theory or technique has been subjected to peer review and publication; (3) in respect to a technique, the error rate and standards for performing the technique are known; and (4) the theory or technique enjoys general acceptance within the relevant scientific community (*Daubert v. Merrell Dow Pharmaceuticals, Inc* 1993). Additionally, the *Daubert* standard established the role of the judge as a "gatekeeper" for the admissibility of scientific evidence, requiring trial courts to scrutinize the reliability of expert evidence (Cheng and Yoon 2005), while *Kumbro Tire Co. v. Carmichael* (1999) later clarified that the *Daubert* criteria are applied to all proposed expert testimony (*Kumho Tire Co. v. Carmichael* 1999).

Notably, legal scholars argue persuasively that there is little additional judicial scrutiny of medical and scientific evidence following the *Daubert* decision (Cheng and Yoon 2005; Kaufman 2001). For example, studies of appellate court decisions show that increased judicial scrutiny of medical expert testimony is the exception, rather than the rule (Shuman 2001). In fact, some state courts have held that "*Daubert* neither requires nor empowers trial courts to determine which of the several competing scientific theories have the best provenance. It demands only that the proponent of the evidence show the [expert testimony] has been arrived at in a scientifically sound and methodologically reliable fashion" (*DiPetrillo v. Dow Chemical Co* 1999).

As the discussion of breach demonstrates, defining the standard of care and the role of expert testimony is intimately linked and unique in medical malpractice tort law. Although physicians are afforded the legal privilege of defining their own standard of care, the process required to define this standard is complex and at times cumbersome in the current legal framework of *Daubert*.

7.4.3 Causation

The next step in the medical malpractice tort law analysis is determining whether a plaintiff has met the evidentiary burden to prove a *causal* nexus between the defendant's negligent behavior and the injury alleged (*Pfiffner v. Correa* 1994). This causation requirement means that a physician's departure from the standard of care alone does not make the case for an injured patient. Rather, the plaintiff must establish facts from which a jury could reasonably conclude that the defendant's actions were a substantial factor in bringing about the harm (*Hamil v. Bashline* 1978). Generating this evidence base, of course, generally relies on expert medical testimony to inform the causation inquiry (*Lyons v. McCauley* 1998).

There are two elements of causation that must be satisfied to succeed in the causation analysis: cause in fact and proximate cause (*Moning v. Alfono* 1977). The plaintiff meets the "cause in fact" burden by demonstrating that "but for" the defendant's actions, the plaintiff's injury would not have occurred (Prosser and Keeton 1984). This requires establishing specific facts to support a reasonable inference of a logical sequence of cause and effect (*Craig ex rel. Craig v. Oakwood Hosp* 2004). The "proximate cause" element is not reached until the plaintiff has satisfied the "cause in fact" burden, and the analysis involves examining the foreseeability of consequences and whether a defendant should be held legally responsible for such consequences (*Skinner v. Square D Co* 1994).

Proximate cause is an elusive concept in tort law. The intent of this element of the causation analysis is to limit the reach of liability and damage payments that flow from negligent behavior (*Derdiarian v. Felix Contr Co* 1980). Generally, the plaintiff meets the burden for proximate cause by showing that the defendant's negligence was a "substantial cause" of the injurious events (*Nallan v. Helmsley-Spear, Inc* 1980), although the relevant case law on this topic is highly variable. This variability is a reflection of the myriad factual circumstances that the "proximate cause" element of tort law must confront both inside and outside the medical malpractice tort law arena.

7.5 Medical Malpractice Tort Law: Justification

Having discussed the process and substance of medical malpractice tort law, it is important to now consider the justifications for this common law regulatory system: compensation and deterrence. The compensatory goal is to restore the injured party to their pre-injury state, while the deterrent goal is to minimize future negligent health care through the threat of civil litigation (Stimson et al. 2010). In the setting of medical malpractice tort law, the compensatory goal could be described as a mechanism of social insurance or the transfer of societal wealth to negligently injured patients, while the deterrent feature provides the means for judicially mediated healthcare quality improvement (Danzon 1985). This dichotomy is important because it provides a framework for measuring the performance of the US healthcare system as a whole, while also providing targets for medical malpractice reform.

Conclusion

The US medical malpractice tort law system is complex. Distinctions between findings of fact and law are critical in understanding the process required to navigate the system, while the role of professional self-regulation, the standard of care, and expert witness testimony illuminates the policy justifications behind the substance of medical malpractice tort law. Finally, the compensatory and deterrent justifications for the system provide a means for both measurement and reform.

References

Alvarez v. Prospect Hosp (1986) NY 2d: NY: Court of Appeals. p 320

Black HC (1999) Black's law dictionary: Kartindo.com

Brunet E (1988) Use and misuse of expert testimony in summary judgment. UC Davis Law Rev 22:93

Chang YC, Eisenberg T, Li TH, Wells MT (2014) Pain and suffering damages in personal injury cases: an empirical study: working paper, New York

Cheng EK, Yoon AH (2005) Does Frye or Daubert matter? A study of scientific admissibility standards. Virginia Law Rev 91:471–513

Church v. Perales (2000) SW 3d: Tenn: Court of Appeals. p 149

Craig ex rel. Craig v. Oakwood Hosp (2004) NW 2d: Mich: Supreme Court. p 296

Danzon PM (1985) Medical malpractice: theory, evidence, and public policy. Harvard University Press, Cambridge

Darby v. Union Planters National Bank of Memphis (1969) SW 2d: Tenn: Supreme Court. p 439

Daubert v. Merrell Dow Pharmaceuticals, Inc. (1993) US: Supreme Court. p 579

Derdiarian v. Felix Contr Co (1980) NY 2d: NY: Court of Appeals. p 308

DiPetrillo v. Dow Chemical Co (1999) A 2d: RI: Supreme Court. p 677

Fay v. Grand Strand Regional Medical Center, LLC (2015) SC: Court of Appeals

Fein v. Permanente Medical Group (1985) P 2d: Cal: Supreme Court. p 665

Franklin MA, Rabin RL (2006) Tort law and alternatives: cases and materials. Foundation Press, New York

Frye v. United States (1923) F: Court of Appeals, Dist. of Columbia. p 1013

Greer v. Advantage Health (2014) NW 2d: Mich: Court of Appeals. p 198

Hamil v. Bashline (1978) A 2d: Pa: Supreme Court. p 1280

Havighurst CC, Blumstein JF, Brennan TA (1998) Health care law and policy: readings, notes, and questions. Foundation Press, New York

Hightower-Warren v. Silk (1997) A 2d: Pa: Supreme Court. p 52

Hodgson v. Bigelow (1939) A 2d. p 338

Jennings v. Case (1999) SW 3d: Tenn: Court of Appeals, Middle Section. p 625

Kaufman H (2001) The expert witness. Neither Frye nor Daubert solved the problem: what can be done? Sci Justice 41(1):7–20

Kelley v. Middle Tenn. Emergency Physicians (2004) SW 3d: Tenn: Supreme Court. p 587

Komlodi v. Picciano (2014) A 3d: NJ: Supreme Court. p 1234

Kumho Tire Co. v. Carmichael (1999) US: Supreme Court. p 137

Lownsbury v. VanBuren (2002) Ohio St 3d: Ohio: Supreme Court. p 231

Lyons v. McCauley (1998) AD 2d: NY: Appellate Div., 2nd Dept. p 516

Maxwell v. Cole (1984) Misc 2d: NY: Supreme Court. p 597

McCoid AH (1958) Care required of medical practitioners. Vand L Rev 12:549

McCullough v. Hutzel Hospital (1979) NW 2d: Mich: Court of Appeals. p 569

McGuckin v. Smith (1992) F 2d: Court of Appeals, 9th Circuit. p 1050

Moning v. Alfono (1977) NW 2d: Mich: Supreme Court. p 759

Moskovitz v. Mt. Sinai Med. Ctr (1994) Ohio St 3d: Ohio: Supreme Court. p 638

Mozingo v. Pitt County Memorial Hosp., Inc. (1992) SE 2d: NC: Supreme Court. p 341

Nallan v. Helmsley-Spear, Inc. (1980) NY 2d: NY: Court of Appeals. p 507

Pedrick v. Peoria & Eastern RR Co (1967) NE 2d: Ill: Supreme Court. p 504

Pfiffner v. Correa (1994) So 2d: La: Supreme Court. p 1228

Preston v. Murty (1987) Ohio St 3d: Ohio: Supreme Court. p 334

Prosser WL, Keeton P (1984) Prosser and Keeton on torts. West Publishing, St. Paul

Regan LJ (1956) Doctor and patient and the law. Am J Med Sci 232(5):602

Seffert v. Los Angeles Transit Lines (1961) Cal 2d: Cal: Supreme Court. p 498

Shuman DW (2001) Expertise in law, medicine, and health care. J Health Polit Policy Law 26(2):267–90

Skinner v. Square D Co (1994) NW 2d: Mich: Supreme Court. p 475

Stimson CJ, Dmochowski R, Penson DF (2010) Health care reform 2010: a fresh view on tort reform. J Urol 184(5):1840–6

Studdert DM, Mello MM, Brennan TA (2004) Medical malpractice. N Engl J Med 350(3):283–92

The pleading and demurrer problems re-examined – new proposals in New York (1960) Columbia Law Rev 60:1015–1034

York v. Rush-Presbyterian-St. Luke's (2006) NE 2d: Ill: Supreme Court. p 635

Systemic Coaching of Staff as Risk Management Tool

8

Regine Töpfer

Abstract

Medicine is a classical team-playing process. Therefore team communication of all staff members is mandatory for successful treatment. However, working together is not given generally.

This chapter shows how coaching of staff is successful in reducing risks.

8.1 Introduction

High Reliability Organizations always had to deal with potentially high-risk situations. They are extreme examples of anticipatory mindful engagement with the unexpected. (Gebauer and Kiel-Dixon 2009)

Medical clinics and practices, which must ensure the highest level of protection and guarantee survival and healing to its patients, can also be considered as High Reliability Organizations (HRO) in the above sense.

As in any context where humans make choices and act on them, human error can lead to injury to persons in this setting as well. In this environment, medical institutions are examining their own failure management with increasing scrutiny. Included herein are the ways in which the "culture of blame" (Chap. 1) can impact the failure quota. This then raises the question, in the communication and interaction between administration, doctors, and nurses, supervisors and employees, and medical personnel and patients, as to which behavior patterns in dealing with one another can lead to catastrophic failures, and on the other hand which behavior patterns can minimize risk of failure to the largest extent (Wehkamp 2010).

In order to allow quality processes and safety instruments such as Critical Incidents Reporting Systems (CIRS), Six Sigma, etc. (Chaps. 6 and 9) to unfold their effectiveness satisfactorily, an organization needs leadership figures and employees who respond to critical incidents as well as actual failures in a constructive fashion, and *together* they need to foster a culture of anticipatory mindfulness when dealing with risks and failures (Gebauer and Kiel-Dixon 2009, p. 44).

Which preconditions to consider and to create in order to foster such a culture, and how human interactions ensue, is covered in Chap. 3. Hospitals and practices as HROs can learn from other HROs. In this context, Gebauer

R. Töpfer, MA
Executive Coach, Rehnocken 67,
Witten 58456, Germany
e-mail: mail@regine-toepfer.de

© Springer-Verlag Berlin Heidelberg 2016
W. Merkle (ed.), *Risk Management in Medicine*, DOI 10.1007/978-3-662-47407-5_8

and Kiel-Dixon describe High Reliability Organizations that have benefited from the strategies and perspectives of the systemic approach:

> Successful HROs attentively pursue anomalies and the smallest of surprises and evaluate these with inquisitiveness. Mistakes are not hastily viewed as an unwanted disturbance caused by human error, but are welcomed as a valuable source of information about the system ("Kaizen", –> Chap. 6). Mistakes reveal a great deal about how the entire system is functioning. How the problem evolved is of greater interest than who could be blamed.
>
> (…) To be attentive to failure, HROs do not only rely on employees' or manager's individual behavior and capacity to act as a role model. Instead, they institutionalize certain practices, observational criteria, etc. to foster a blame-free culture and to encourage mindful behavior. (Gebauer and Kiel-Dixon 2009, p. 42)

8.2 Systemic Organizational Development

While in biology and somatic medicine the term "systemic" concerns the organism and its environment, systemic organizational development relates to complex social systems.

In this context, systemic organizational theory contrasts with traditional organizational administrative theories that describe an "organization as a multidimensional social system, which, while having a life of its own, can and does only exist by being a subsystem of larger systems" (Table 8.1) (Königswieser and Hillebrand 2009, S. 30f.).

Table 8.1 Multidimensional organization

Organizations	
According to business-centric organizational theory	According to systemic organizational theory
…are designed in a goal-oriented, deliberate and rational way	…are complex and dynamic
…enable rational purposeful action	…are ambivalent and contradictive
	…are processual and conflict-prone

In the systemic approach to risk management, one adapts a mindful and curious view of things, which results in the ability to respond in a swift and flexible manner. These qualities require, on an individual as well as interpersonal level, certain attitudes in the following areas:

Perception
Mindfulness and curiosity are to be understood as a wakeful awareness, which is occurring in a situation. Focused on the present moment, this awareness sharpens ones perception as to the qualities of the processes, as well as the related communications and interactions among those involved.

Recognition
Recognition, when perceived as genuine, can be a source of motivation and energy for the recipient. Which levels of perception constitute an informed recognition is described by Zwack et al. (2011 p. 432+) as follows:

1. Level of explicit recognition of physical presence (observing common courtesy rules)
2. Level of recognition of performance within the boundaries of a specific professional role or job function, through honest praise and constructive criticism (Here recognition means "estimation of value.")
3. Level of respecting personal values ("An employee wants to be taken seriously in his professional capacity, but not be mistaken for it.")

Communication
Especially in fundamental organizational change processes which affect employee procedures as well as their behavior patterns, the participants can no longer fall back on their habitual routines. Mindfulness and recognition/appreciation will ensure a continued, if not clearly improved, flow of information. In some cases where well-placed feedback in critical situations is designed to steer things back

on course, it may be necessary to disregard strict established hierarchies. This however is only possible if the respect offered is genuine and not just derived from hierarchical circumstances.

Beyond this, repetition of mistakes can be markedly reduced by engaging all involved, and possibly also external observers, in a comprehensive review of which processes and behaviors lead to a negative result, "with the goal of learning as much as possible about the systemic relationships" (Gebauer and Kiel-Dixon 2009, p. 42), and from there derive the necessary fundamental changes for the future.

8.3 Transformation of Organizational Culture

Due to the necessity of introducing risk management, the resulting targeted changes in behavioral patterns and communication strategies, and the deliberately guided implementation of new organizational strategies and goals, the medical organizations are undergoing a cultural transformation.

Beyond this, the generational differences of the last several decades are fundamentally presenting organizations with challenges.

Table 8.2 attempts to emphasize the change in generational values, which has led to a change in perception of leadership and hierarchy, and will – in coming years – continue to have far-reaching impact.

In medical circles and elsewhere, the "demands of the Millennials" (Klaffke and Becker 2012) is a hot topic for discussion:

> "Are They Willing to Work Too?" reads the polemic title of an article in the newspaper "Die Zeit". "But studies have not shown that Generation Y is less productive: In a 2010 youth study by Shell the qualities of industriousness and ambition were high on the list. More people than ever are receiving high school diplomas, and they study more efficiently and with more goal-orientation. (…) 'Can't be bothered' is no longer a familiar expression these days. The resumes of these young talents are filled with internships, courses, trips abroad and social engagement. The Ys aren't just demanding of their employers, they expect much of themselves as well. (Bund et al. 2013)

Because several generations in different hierarchy levels usually work together in a clinic, divergent needs and expectations need to be brought into harmony. Peak performance is often achieved where the personal effort is done with engagement and motivation. This can only happen if in the collaboration the basic values in regard to the different professional roles and functions can be assured. In this context, the mutual appreciation achieved through open feedback takes on special importance:

> The idealistic expectations of generation Y will suffer a blow in some ways; the employers on the other hand will have to learn to think more creatively in order to motivate those smart young minds and to keep their attention. In this sense, the current state of the job market offers perhaps the best opportunity for both sides to get to know each other, and to initiate the process of adapting. (Barth and Lambsdorff 2009)

Table 8.2 Different skills in different generations

Skill	Baby boomer (*1955–1965)	Generation X (*1965–1979)	Generation Y (*1980–2000)
Problem-solving	Hierarchical	Independently, self-reliantly	Within the group
Mastering tasks	Sequentially	Multitasking as needed	Multitasking as a given
Communication	Centered around hierarchical structures	Centered around personal relationships	Interconnected and transparent
Leadership style	Hierarchical	Collaboration with subordinates	Based on partnership
Feedback	Annually or biannually	Monthly or weekly	Upon request, "open-door", mentoring
Decision making	Independently, team is informed	Independently, while also considering team's opinions	By consensus, during discussion with the team

The leaders in any organization are the ones who bear the responsibility of transforming the company culture: as the initiators of such change (Vision, Values, Strategy), as positive role models for the entire team, and through a confident, situationally appropriate leadership style that is attuned to the individuality of their employees. Because cultural change cannot be simply "decreed" in a top-down manner, executives are "dependent upon comprehending, actively shaping, and adapting responsibility for relatively autonomous units and their key players, and upon the intertwining of independently running processes. Highly qualified independent units don't need fewer leaders, but better ones" (Schmid and Messmer 2005, p. 209).

In this sense, executives must achieve effectiveness through their own behavior, by not just demanding, but also fostering the desired new behaviors, the development of the pertinent skills, the acceptance of the company values, and the identification with the intended company goals.

However, executives in healthcare organizations rarely learn enough about these skills essential for a successful leadership. Since the medical world is gaining in complexity, demanding that besides the medical knowledge itself, one must develop knowledge of such things as operating efficiency and profitability in order to gain a position such as head physician; (future) executives need to receive further training. In most cases this takes place in parallel to doing the core work of leading a clinic/department, if at all. With coaching, this continuing training can be successfully and effectively tackled.

8.4   Executive Coaching

Coaching supports executives in:

- Mobilizing the willingness to change in regard to the urgent necessity of a new organizational culture
- The development of new perspectives, attitudes, and routines
- The handling of emotions in the process (stress management)

- Reflecting on the leadership role and leadership style, respectively
- Developing authentic and appropriate ways of communicating and interacting that are in keeping with the organizational culture
- The realignment and goal setting of individual executives and entire teams

Team as well as individual coaching focuses on the person, i.e., individuals in their professional roles, and on the ways in which they deal with change. Here the coachee's stance relative to the customer differs fundamentally from the "traditional" stance of the adviser or even the doctor.

Comparison of different customer demands and respective attitudes of the service provider (after Radatz 2003, p. 88+) is as follows:

1. Demand of customer from the expert (advisor): "The problem is for YOU to take on, and for YOU to solve!"
2. Demand of patient from the doctor: "YOU need to tell me where/what my problem is (1), then YOU need to take it on (2) and YOU need to solve it for me (3)!"
3. Demand of coachee from the coach: "Your role is to help ME recognize where my problem lies, and support me in MY resulting resolution attempts!"

In the coaching process, through questioning techniques and other tools from systemic change work, the coach ensures a solutions-oriented process and the return to the customer's resources. This helps the coachee to avoid the downward spiral of problem- and weakness-centric thinking and to leave the problem space behind in favor of constructive changes in the solution space.

> Problem space is not solution space. (Albert Einstein)

> Resource-focus, solution-focus, customer-focus

> These three terms are closely related. They describe basic attitudes of systemic practices: To think resourcefully, to move toward concrete solutions, and to consistently have the customer's interests in mind. […] Central to this is the assumption that each system already inherently possesses the

resources necessary to solve its own problems – it is just not using them at that time. In order to unearth these resources, one need not occupy oneself (at least not intensively) with the problem, the focus lies with the creation of solutions from the very start. (Schlippe and Schweitzer 2012, p. 209)

In this sense, the encounters in the context of coaching occur among equals and apply to the relationship between the coach and customer (e.g., clinic leadership) as well as between the coach and coachee (e.g., chief resident). For the customer's success, it is imperative that not only are all involved taken seriously in their respective areas of expertise but that they also adopt self-responsibility in the process – this is illustrated below via the task clarification.

8.5 Solutions-Oriented Change Work

As early as the 1970s Watzlawick, Weakland, and Fisch formulated the four underlying steps of solutions-oriented change work (Walker 2004, p. 246):

1. Clear and concrete problem definition
2. Examination of failed solution attempts
3. Clear goal (solution) definition
4. Formulation and execution of a plan to bring about this solution

While step 4 is part of the coaching process itself, steps 1–3 comprise a comprehensive goal and task clarification as the beginning of the coaching process. The field of tension between the demands of an organization (company mission) and the needs of individual personalities require a precise handling of complex issues.

Goal and task clarification contributes substantially to the success of coaching through:

- Concrete, clearly defined goals and subgoals
- Concrete, clearly defined time frame
- Clarification and honoring of the roles of all involved in the change process
- Separating which developmental goals shall be achieved via coaching and which shall be achieved by other means

- Implementing feedback loops
- Clarification of the developmental processes' parameters for the organization itself as well as for the coaching process

Based on Schlippe and Schweitzer (2012, pp. 235), we differentiate between *four different phases of task clarification*:

1. Impetus
2. Objective
3. Task
4. Offer

This is illustrated via the example of individual coaching for an executive:

- Impetus (Status Quo)
- The focus on the safety of patients requires the introduction of comprehensive risk management. The executive leadership becomes shapers of a new leadership culture in the organization and thereby is supported in the change process by individual coaching.
- Objective (Target State)
  - Definition of organization objectives (error rate approaching zero).
  - The concrete and detailed definition of the skills to be acquired or expanded, which are necessary for reaching the goal and which shall characterize the communication and interaction (culture) of the organization in the future.
  - The concrete roles that shall be played by executives and employees. This clarifies for the participants their place in the overall process, as well as the concrete context of the measures to be taken.
- Assignment of Tasks
  - By the Supervisor to the Executive
    This concerns the executive's concrete developmental goals that impact their role, i.e., their professional personality, for example, the definition of leadership role and style, identification with these qualities, and the dos and don'ts of leadership in the context of the desired organizational culture.

– By the Supervisor to the Coach

The supervisor clarifies the expectations he has about the coach's professional conduct. The goals that were discussed with the executive are elucidated. As in the discussion with the employee, the supervisor makes clear how he will notice that the employee is on the right path during the process and that he has finally reached his goal.

– By the Coachee to the Coach

As the real coaching begins, the coach learns from the executive in a one-by-one discussion, which concrete changes they have set as a goal for themselves. The task as such (in terms of content) is by the coachee to the coach. Then they work out every detail of this contract. The prerequisite for this is that in the preliminary stages of the coaching, the organizational contract between the supervisor and employee has been worked out as concretely as possible!

• Presentation of Offer

The tasks on the side of the company vs. the employees differ in their organizational perspectives as well as their degree of concreteness. Accordingly, the coach makes two offers:

1. On the company level, the offer relates to the goal of the organization as a whole.
2. On the coaching level, the offer relates to the personal goals that the executive derives from point 1 for their professional development.

During the clarification of the offers, the coach not only makes his methods transparent but also examines the various task details as to their ambitiousness and feasibility.

8.6   Implementing New Forms of Communication

In the framework of the cultural transformation, the task clarification ensures that the communication between the participants gets started in a purposeful way. Thus the result is not solely the arrival at a coaching goal via the coachee. Another result is that through the process of task clarification, a new of communication is implemented, as it relates to

• Flow of information
• Feedback loops
• Clarity of roles
• Clarity of goals
• Precise joint shaping of the future

The following fundamental aspects of communication should be practiced by the supervisor during the task clarification with this employee:

• Empathy – goal orientation

The supervisor needs to be open and available to his employee right from the start of the task clarification and needs to focus not only on their developmental goals but also the resources that the employee already inherently has at his disposal. These inherent resources form the raw materials with which the desired development will take place.

The supervisor should focus on the skills and qualifications, which the executive brings to the table for the planned development and mentions them with concrete examples. Through the supervisor's detailed positive feedback, the executive can become aware of previously undiscovered resources (as a rule one can assume that the problem awareness is distinctly more present than the solution awareness). And he can perceive and register the information as an appreciation of his person. This not only strengthens the level of relationship between the supervisor and employee but also guides the employee methodically toward solutions- and resource-oriented thinking from the very start.

• Pacing: Leading
• The supervisor builds on the employee's experience as well as his needs (pacing), to make coaching plausible and attractive as a new methodology.

The employee receives all information necessary for him to recognize that coaching is based on trust and is tailored to him, the customer.

The supervisor imparts his own (meta-)perspectives on the developmental process and with that emphasizes the connection between the desired organizational goal and the employee's personal development (leading).

- Dealing with Mutual Expectations

At this point in the process, one must become aware of expectations on different levels. Schlippe and Schweitzer explain about the interaction of mutual expectations:

A person forms expectations about the things that others expect from them. And since a person is never an island to themselves, these expectations of expectations belonging to the various members of a system tend to intertwine and form patterns […]. (Schlippe and Schweitzer 2010, p. 12)

Therefore we want to implement feedback loops between the participants:

1. How does the employee value the supervisor's feedback as it relates to his developmental potential?
2. How does the employee value the coaching methods? What expectations does he believe the coach has of him?
3. What is the employee's motivation for change (intrinsically/extrinsically)?
4. What would need to be ensured for the employee in order for them to feel comfortable saying "no" to the coaching (or the coach)?

8.7 Positioning the Participants in the Change Process

The task clarification process also clarifies the positioning of all participants in the change process itself and makes the process transparent at this point. What comes into view here as well is which individual thought and behavior patterns support the change process, which thought and behavior patterns disrupt the process, and – in this context especially important – which resistances may arise, if any.

As an example, such a change process can be the introduction of a risk management system at a clinic or practice. By facilitating this change process, external coaching offers the customer a safe space in which he can deal with his concerns in a solutions-oriented way. Here concerns are understood as themes to be mindful of, themes that have up to now been neglected or consciously blocked out, because they didn't seem compatible with the goals of the company or organization at first glance.

Often the concerns that arise in the process of coaching turn out to be pointers to blind spots in the goal setting, which necessitate an adjustment at this point. Beyond this, the concerns of the coachee often bring values to the surface that they must try to bring over into the new company culture as well, so that they may continue their activity in the company with dedication and loyalty.

To this end, systemic coaching equips the customer to

1. Distill the values from ones own concerns
2. Work out ways to assure these values into the future
3. Do this in a way that does justice to both the goal and the customer
4. Actively communicate the resulting solutions throughout the company
5. Therefore strengthen ones own contribution to the cultural transformation

This approach goes hand in hand with the overall picture of events that the executive should stay aware of when looking at their own situation from a meta-level. The coach helps with the process of zooming back and forth between the everyday details and the big picture. Their task is to provide precise and effective tools in this regard.

The key players in the change process have the opportunity, through individual coaching, to view themselves in connection with the company goal. This allows them space to assess their attitude toward the company goal, their motivation, as well as their room for maneuver.

A change process that does not provide this space for reflection remains too general, because it cannot meet the ones who hold key functions individually.

References

Barth LJ, Lambsdorff M (2009) Talent Management. Werben um die Generation Y [Talent Management. Wooing Generation Y]. How to attract, nurture, and retain this confident and demanding new generation of talent employees. Fokus 70–73

Bund K, Heuser UJ, Kunze A (2013) Wollen Die Auch Arbeiten? [Are they willing to work too?] Die Zeit 23–24. 3/11/2013

Gebauer A, Kiel-Dixon U (2009) Das Nein zur eigenen Wahrnehmung ermoeglichen [Gaining the ability to say no to one's own perceptions]. Handling extreme situations through building organisational skills. Organisational development. Zeitschrift fuer Unternehmensentwicklung und Change Management, Heft 3, pp 40–49

Klaffke M, Becker KA (2012) Personal management im Krankenhaus: Die Ansprüche der "Millennials". Deutsches Ärzteblatt, S, A1020-A1022

Königswieser R, Hillebrand M (2009) Einführung in die systemische Organisationsberatung. [Systemic consultancy in organisations]. Carl Auer, Heidelberg

Lehky M (2011) Leadership 2.0: Wie Führungskräfte die neuen Herausforderungen im Zeitalter von Smartphone, Burnout & Co. managen... [How executives can rise to the new challenges in the age of Smartphones, Burnout, and Co.. ...]. Campus Verlag, Springer, p 113

Radatz S (2003) Beratung ohne Ratschlag. Systemisches Coaching für Führungskräfte und BeraterInnen. [Consulting without advice: system coaching for executives and consultants]. Systemisches Management, Wien

Schlippe A v., Schweitzer J (2010) Systemische interventionen [Systemic interventions]. Vandenhoeck & Ruprecht, Göttingen

Schlippe A v., Schweitzer J (2012) Lehrbuch der systemischen Therapie und Beratung I. Das Grundlagenwissen [Textbook of systemic therapy and counseling]. Vandenhoeck & Ruprecht, Göttingen

Schmid B, Messmer A (2005) Systemische Personal-, Organisations- und Kulturentwicklung. Konzepte und Perspektiven [Systemic development of human resources, organisation and culture]. EHP – Verlag Andreas Kohlhage, Bergisch-Gladbach

Walker W (2004) Abenteuer Kommunikation. Bateson, Persl, Satir, Erickson und die Anfänge des Neurolinguistischen Programmierens (NLP) [The adventure of communication. Bateson, Persl, Satir, Erickson and the Beginnings of Neurolinguistic Programming (NLP)]. Klett-Cotta, Stuttgart

Wehkamp K-H (2010) Fehlverhalten – zwischen Fürsorge und Machtausübung [Misconduct – between care and exercise of power]. In: Borgwart J, Kolpatzik K (eds) Aus Fehlern lernen – Fehlermanagement in Gesundheitsberufen [Learning from errors – failure management in the health professions]. Springer, Heidelberg, pp 89–98

Zwack M, Muraitis A, Schweitzer-Rothers J (2011) Wozu keine Wertschätzung? Zur Funktion des Wertschätzungsdefizits in Organisationen [The function of the lack of appreciation in organizations]. Online-Publikation 04. 11/2011, Verlag für Sozialwissenschaften

Sigrid Blehle

Abstract

CIRS means: luckily a mistake has not led to injury of a patient, but this almost mistake is a source of improvement avoiding such situation again. Details of the CIRS process are pointed out.

In a clinic corporation with several hospitals of different levels of medical care, it is mandatory to consider risk management in different directions from the side of patient care as well as operational and required by law management of quality and risk required by law.

(The principles of CIRS prescribed in this chapter are the same in single organized hospitals.)

9.1 CIRS as Element of Clinical Risk Management

In a clinical group, the main purpose is to treat patients optimally in every single hospital and to create a trustful and secure environment for patients and employees.

Frame of clinical risk management is defined through:

- Ethical principles in medicine (i.e., code of medical ethics, constitution, Hippocratic Oath, etc.)
- Medical liability law
- Common legislation
- Institutions (WHO Collaborating Centre for Patient Safety, "Aktionsbündnis Patientensicherheit")

In a hospital group, CIRS (critical incident reporting system) should be oriented toward the CIRS concept of St. Gallen which is recommended by Aktionsbündnis Patientensicherheit e.V. Critical events should be detected and

S. Blehle, MD, MBA
Managing Partner, Köhn und Kollegen,
Widenmayerstr. 34, Munich 80538, Germany
e-mail: sblehle@gmx.de

© Springer-Verlag Berlin Heidelberg 2016
W. Merkle (ed.), *Risk Management in Medicine*, DOI 10.1007/978-3-662-47407-5_9

eliminated as soon as possible. To guarantee patients' security during treatment on continuous high-level potential, existing sources of hazard will be detected and eliminated; see Chap. 11.

The setup of a culture of security in which promotive safety behavior boosts itself is the main target.

Principles of CIRS are:

- No sanctions
- Confidentiality and anonymity
- Analysis by experts
- Information and response with preservation of confidentiality and anonymity
- Defined processes and responsibilities with transparent ways of communication and of handling
- Fairness
- Support by management
- Data security

- Principle of clients, i.e., that every hospital only administrate their own reports, and such reports are released explicitly through other hospitals and which are imported through central structures of the group.

Necessary instruments for implementing CIRS are special CIRS concept, defined CIRS workgroup in every hospital, involvement of concern-wide employee organization, and a simply usable software tool, which can also connect and analyze informations. A concern-wide employment agreement should be the result of early coordination with concern-wide employee organization. Through this agreement, CIRS is established formally for all employees.

Structures which are implemented in context with CIRS have to support this. These can look, e.g., like the following structures:

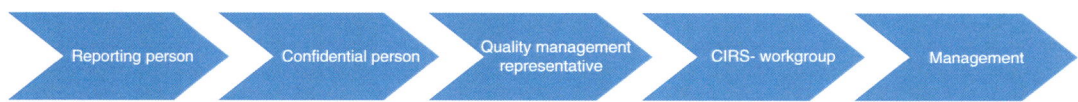

A secure anonymous report is of maximum importance. If e-mail reporting would be used, obvious confidential reporting is impossible. In this case, strong legislation of data security has to be implemented prior to CIRS activation.

At present, it is a further problem that CIRS data could be confiscated through prosecution. In the case of e-mail, this can relatively simply lead to subsequent personalization of the CIRS report followed by punishing. This legal problem (q.v. Chap. 1) has to be solved. But this is not in the hands of a single hospital or enterprise.

It is also an alternative that a CIRS report is paper based and can be thrown anonymously into a special postbox. So traceability is nearly excluded.

The management and the CIRS process group decide together which improvements will be implemented in current business and which will be communicated across the group. So other hospitals of the group can benefit from these. (A single organized hospital can join peer groups of public hospital organizations.)

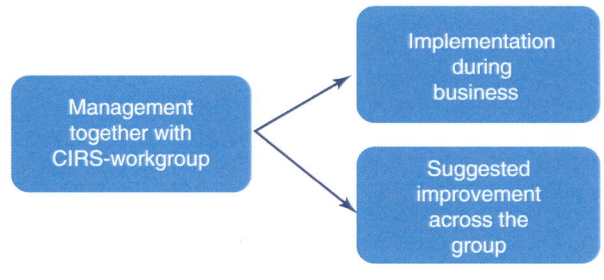

Development of confidence inside the organization and accentuation of the importance by the responsible management are absolute requirements for successful implementation of CIRS. It is very important that CIRS will be carried out from all performance levels of the enterprise.

Implementation of CIRS serves especially for improving of quality of organizational structures and processes and thus continuously improving patient care. This is supported through knowledge transfer and analysis round tables across the group. So it is possible to eradicate mistakes company-wide and to avoid critical incidents. CIRS is an important part of the continuous improvement process.

Of every CIRS announcement there is an additional benefit if it is been evident in every single hospital.

In private practices, CIRS is usually unnecessary because organization is relatively small and transparent so that mistakes or nearly mistakes are known. In a large medical practice with several doctors, introduction of CIRS is also useful.

In such a case, this private practice can use CIRS assistance of professional associations. On the other hand, a hospital will always create their own CIRS system. But the principles are naturally always the same.

executive board, supervisory board, and auditors. Furthermore, setup of risk management is required by law. KonTraG concerns not only stock corporations. Also limited joint-stock partnership (KGaA) and many limiteds (Ltd., GmbH) have to implement this, especially if there is a supervisory committee with worker participation or a facultative supervisory committee. Additionally, there are guidelines of Basel II, which oblige banks for individual risk rating of enterprises financed through them, the necessary of corporate risk management as part of corporate governance.

In Section 91 paragraph 2 of Aktiengesetz (AktG), there is verbally prescribed that "the board of directors has to prepare appropriate arrangements e.g. implementation of a system of monitoring so that developments, which will threat the continued existence of the organization, are detected early". Additionally, auditors are obliged to check the new regulations especially in respect to existence and operating of a risk management system and related arrangements in the area of intern auditing and to make it to part of auditor's report.

More or less, these measures are similar in all developed countries. For European and US law details, please refer to the specific chapters.

9.2   Corporate Risk Management

Usage of corporate risk management is the consequence of the guidelines of the so-called law for control and transparence in corporate division (KonTraG: Gesetz zur Kontrolle und Transparenz im Unternehmensbereich). In this law, extension of liability is determined on the

9.3   Summary

In a clinical corporation, clinical risk management is closely connected with economically risk management. Here, management of mistakes on basis of CIRS is an important part of risk prophylaxis. Therefore, all groups like patients, employees, and payers will get their benefits.

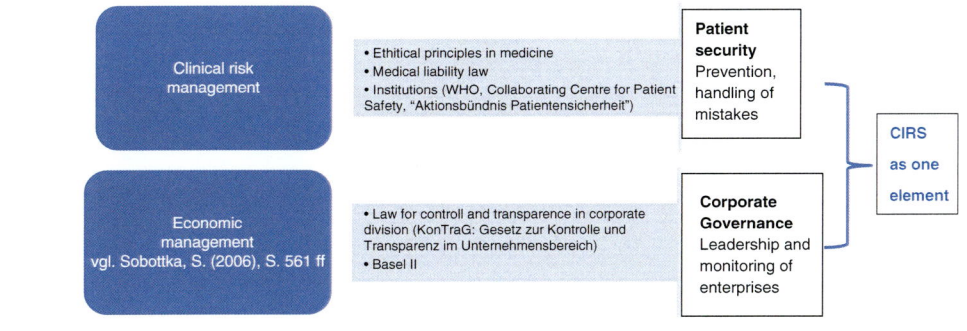

It is very important, that these cases will be handled systematically and that these informations will be used across the group and will be connected together. Result is a learning process of the complete concern. It is mandatory that every employee get access to knowledge out of the workup of CIRS cases.

Bigger corporations need more necessary an automatical CIRS reporting system then smaller ones to gain important lessons learned.

Results herefrom on the following levels are:

Ideally, this leads across the group to sustainable avoidance of such critical situations across

- Management level:
  - Role model function
  - Definition of in-house responsibilities
  - Offer of continued education in reference to improvement and development of safety-relevant behavior

the group and to enhancement of patient security. Simultaneously, incorrect behavior and possible emergent right of liability will be reduced through this learning process (Chaps. 15, 20).

- Individual level:
  - Self-reflecting scrutinizing basic attitude
  - Careful and cautious acting

Walter Merkle

Abstract

Communication is a principal tool to solve complex challenges, e.g. avoiding mistakes. However, there are situations which are very sensitive, thus communication can cause failures. Therefore, it is important to know under which circumstances communication is working in which manner.

Observational Teamwork Assessment for Surgery is the description which interactions take place within an OR team during the operation.

As shown during the EAU congress in 2011, interactions in such a team are routine, but unconsciously they can influence the OR result.

Communication is an important tool in risk management and failure prevention.

However, when reading the OTAS study one might develop doubts about the value of communication. The study impressively shows that unnecessary communication was the cause for poor result of the operation, because it negatively influenced the concentration of the surgeon.

The consequence of this realization is that communication at the right place is unrenounceable, but during an operation it has to be limited to the lowest possible level. Unnecessary interruption increases failure rate because it disturbs the concentration of the surgeon and the team members as well.

Due to more and more establishing time shift work, it can happen that longer operations will see change of the OR nurse. Each new team member must be briefed shortly not to break the concentration of the entire team.

Therefore it can be wise to better organize the OR team to reduce such disruptions, which might increase failure rate.

The OTAS study observed teams of general surgery and urology. There was no difference (development, initial reliability and validity testing of an observational tool for assessing technical skills of operation room nurses). Therefore the perception of this study is general (Sevdalis et al. 2009).

Consequence: Operations need full concentration, although statistically, all human beings do something wrong almost every minute. Therefore failure during operations can be fatal. Thus it is absolutely mandatory to avoid disrupting the OR team with unnecessary communication so that the surgeon and his team are fully concentrated on their operation procedure.

W. Merkle, MD
Riskmanager in Medicine Specialist in Urology, Management Expert for Hospitals (VWA), German Diagnostic Clinic – Helios Clinic, Aukammallee 33, Wiesbaden D 65191, Germany
e-mail: Risikomanagement.Merkle@hotmail.de

Optimizing communication

Not only is the individual experience and capability important for the result of an operation, but it also depends on the optimized team communication (Undre et al. 2007: OTAS – refinement and application in urological surgery).

During the study a team of supervisors observed a list which contained

- Patient's condition
- Equipment (by hand; complete?)
- Communication behavior (necessary/unnecessary, cooperation, coordination, team leading, monitoring)

Poor teamwork led to numerous failures and later poor healing.

The complexity and coordination in a team is mirrored in the results.

Task list contents:

- Patient task: individual situation (clotting time, diabetes, cardiac health, former diseases, etc.)
- Equipment and provision tasks: instruments, checklists, tissues are complete at end of operation, etc.
- Communication tasks: OR team, formal consent prior to procedure, patient's details (e.g. x-ray images), other special conditions

The teamwork-related behavior was evaluated as

- Quality of communication (concerning the words needed for the procedure)
- Coordination of team members
- Cooperation of all team members including staff assisting the team from outside
- Leading the operation (surgeon has the right of the last decision but has to pay attention to observations and information of his team members)
- Monitoring (the team takes part actively and informs the surgeon about important things during the procedure)

It is obvious that these kinds of behavior skills are well known in the aviation business.

There, flat hierarchy is standard – and the secret to good results of OR teams. CRM contributes to make a good functioning OR team out of accidentally working staff members as a team.

This is also an aviation technique which is gaining more and more importance especially in big hospitals where teams are not working together constantly but built together from case to case, and where these teams must be able to do even complex surgery in perfect quality without great discussions to come to a common basis. This describes the learning effect from OTAS studies.

There are three main groups of actors:

- Surgeons
- Anesthesiologists
- Nurses

They work together in three periods:

- Pre-operative (main briefing)
- Intra-operative (TTO)
- Post-operative (transfer from OR to ICU, etc.)

In all three of these periods communication is necessary.

Before an operation – similar to before a flight – briefing of the complete team is mandatory.

Thus all staff members – independent of their position and function – must be completely informed and know where the specific problems of the case are. Many things must be drawn to attention, and information is necessary: current condition, clinical risk factors, prior operations, allergy, drug interactions, anatomic variations, complication in former operations, etc. All important things must be pointed out.

Additionally the planned procedure must be described, especially when the operation will be complex.

Intra operatively, communication must be reduced to a minimum, e.g. the normal instructions of the surgeon to his assisting doctor and nurse. In case of an unexpected situation during the running procedure, TTO (see Chap. 12) must be performed so that the team thinks together over the new situation. After a conclusion is made the procedure can continue.

Post operatively, surgeon and anesthesiologist must transfer the patient to the ICU. The transfer of all information from OR to ICU must be complete – as well as the data from the briefing of operation itself.

Why is this so important?

Because everybody, including the surgeon, is capable of making mistakes. Therefore all staff members must contribute and must help the surgeon not to overlook anything so that the procedure itself can be performed without failure.

This is the claim:

Everybody makes mistakes – but the team does not!

Apprenticeship from the OTAS study

The results of the study are as follows:

- Best score was for complete information regarding patient's health status.
- The status of the equipment was irregularly discussed.
- The worst status was quality of team communication.

The lack of information from each other concerning equipment can bring many problems during an operation especially when doing technical operations like MICS (minimally invasive cardiac surgery). MIC does depend on doubtless functioning of the equipment. Even a little dysfunction might risk the success – and therefore the patient's health! Therefore it is mandatory to check the equipment carefully prior to starting the operation. In case there is any problem, all staff members must be informed to find a solution.

This routine check procedure is part of the risk management process.

Example

Defects in OR instruments from the Far East (FR-online 05.08.2011):

- Two-thirds of all OR instruments worldwide come from Sialkot/Pakistan.
- Although Global Players sell the instruments, the quality control in reality is performed in

small garage companies in Sialkot (BBC information).

- CE certification "light" is possible in Rumania.
- Health administration could check the quality coming from abroad but normally does not due to lack of manpower.
- Some of these instruments are produced by children so that cost is reduced.

Therefore it pays to check where instruments are coming from and whether they are produced by children, which would be unacceptable. The lower the price, the greater these risks.

Another big problem is the transfer of patients from one unit to another, e.g. OR to ICU. As the OTAS study shows, there is a lack of information. Most often the surgeon "forgets" to inform the other staff members. Therefore it is wise to organize this transfer accompanied by a transfer protocol to fill out.

It should contain

- Diagnosis
- OR procedure
- Kind of anesthesia
- Complications
- Drugs given/necessary
- Mandatory control procedures: breathing, lab, urine production, etc.

FORDEC is a good tool to transform such experiences from the OTAS study to a successful solution.

Furthermore, the human resources problem has to be addressed. Surgeons especially have to accept that they tend to overestimate their part in an operation. This can lead to overconfidence.

The attitude of pilots helps to prevent mistakes. Doctors can learn a lot from this attitude, because they tend to overestimate themselves and the biological borders, thus failures might occur.

Thus the apprenticeship from the OTAS study is followed by optimizing the behavior in the OR. Briefings are installed and checklists routinely used. However because each hospital is individual these principal tools must be tailored individually for a hospital. This is best done in an interdisciplinary work group led by an experienced moderator.

The goal of all of these actions is to succeed in risk-free treatment of the given patients, who trustfully come into a hospital to get cured.

We are servants and not masters of the patients!

Literature

Postersession 110, EAU Congress Wien (2011)

Sevdalis N, Undre S, Henry J, Sydney E, Koutantji M, Darzi A, Vincent CA: Development, initial reliability and validity testing of an observational tool for assessing technical skills of operating room nurses (2009) Int J Nurs Stud 46(9):1187–1193

Undre S, Sevdalis N, Healey AN, Darzi A, Vincent CA: Observational teamwork assessment for surgery (OTAS): refinement and application in urological surgery (2007) World J Surga

FMEA

Achim Göbel

Abstract

FMEA means that potential failures in the near future are anticipated, thus one can act to avoid them in the reality to come.

The details of successful FMEA process are pointed out.

FMEA (failure mode and effects analysis/ Fehlermöglichkeits- und Einflussanalyse), as a universal method model, follows the basic idea of a preventive avoidance of errors instead of a remedial error detection and correction. Errors are very unlikely to happen when already early considered in the identification and assessment of potential causes in the development of a system or concept. FMEA and FMECA (failure mode and effects analysis and critical analysis) are analytical methods of reliability engineering to identify potential vulnerabilities in advance.

To avoid the consequences of errors, this forward-looking analysis method was developed to discover machine errors at an early stage and hopefully upfront a failure.

It all started in the aerospace industry where forward planning was vital for the astronauts and former pilots.

FMEA then was taken by the auto industry, especially Ford and Toyota, who have developed customized FMEA systems for their enterprises.

In current medicine, FMEA only shows up at medical device manufacturers whereas in the operating rooms or in the treatment of patients, it is still rarely encountered – although, forward planning may prevent complications herein especially. In curative medicine, there is no systematic FMEA except for sporadic attempts in the (most complicated) individual cases.

Avoiding the emergence of incidents is less costly than a regulation or correction of a failure thereafter. In medicine, this usually ends up in a lost liability case (see Chap. 15). As an example, the cost explosion of a delayed error detection is shown in Fig. 11.1.

Types and further development of FMEA.

- System FMEA
- Design FMEA
- Process FMEA
- Machinery FMEA

A. Göbel
AirColleg GmbH, Buchenweg 17,
Weilmünster 35789, Germany
e-mail: info@aircolleg.de

© Springer-Verlag Berlin Heidelberg 2016
W. Merkle (ed.), *Risk Management in Medicine*, DOI 10.1007/978-3-662-47407-5_11

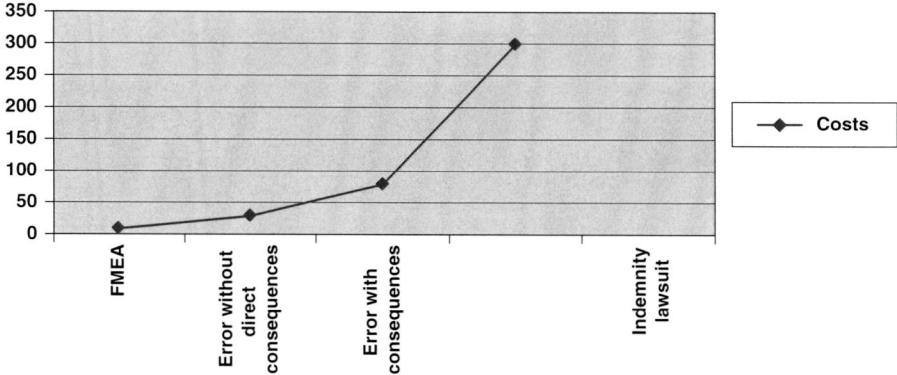

Fig. 11.1 Cost explosion in delayed error detection (Courtesy of AirColleg GmbH)

11.1 System FMEA

The System FMEA examines the interaction of subsystems (different disciplines and departments) in a superior system (e.g., hospital), as well as the interaction of several processes (action sequences) in a complex system. Thereby, it aims to identify potential weak points (error sources) especially at intersections which evolve out of the individual disciplines and departments and also their interactions. The consideration includes random and systematic errors during operation.

As the work of hospitals is getting more complex, it is important to consider these relationships. Figure 11.2 illustrates the chronological sequence of individual actions and their interdependencies.

Basically, upfront a new process, you have to look out in advance for the avoidance of errors and, additionally, that possible random errors are identified early enough.

That means that we have to utilize two parallel FMEA processes that also belong together integrally. Spoken technically, we differentiate between the following FMEA methods:

- Design FMEA
- Process FMEA
- Machinery FMEA

11.2 Design FMEA

Design FMEA aims at the recognition of a changed product and the avoidance of errors which have been already successfully eliminated/avoided in the predecessor system but which may sneak back into the next generation due to redesign(s). To recognize and avoid them prospectively is essential.

In the medical field, a strategy in terms of Microsoft – delivering unfinished software versions to the market and hoping that the "FMEA" is done in arrears by customer criticism – is unthinkable.

The only exception to this is the learning effect in the field of pathology, although dissections are becoming increasingly rare.

In this respect but not systematically, the medical branch tries to avoid treatment errors in general by creating means of SOPs and guidelines. When revising these rules, it is very helpful to consider Design FMEA to take into account already valid and proven information for the new version correctly.

11.3 Process FMEA

Process FMEA is an important tool for hospitals. To think through processes and optimizing the same increase the success of treatments. It reduces the burden on patients, shortens

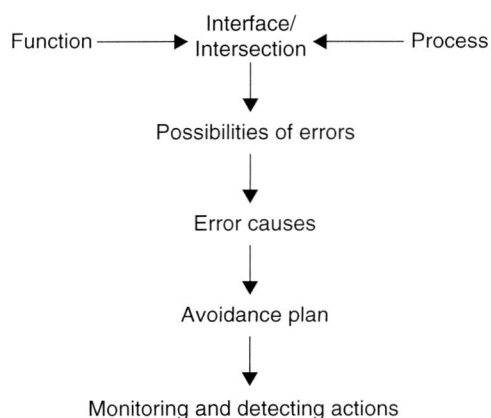

Fig. 11.2 System FMEA – sequence of activities and their dependencies

(without incurring medical compromise) the length of stay, increases patient satisfaction, reduces (without having to save) the costs, and increases the profit of the hospital which may be invested in new equipment and personnel, etc.

In hospitals, Process FMEA can be currently found only rudimentary in simulations of so-called clinical pathways. These are, as far as known, only one-dimensional, i.e., they are aligned for proper medical procedures. While this is essential and fundamental for a Process FMEA, the abovementioned aspects may be integrated easily – a classic win-win situation.

11.3.1 Example: Length of Stay for TURP (Prostate Resection)

When the preoperative safety procedures (lab, ECG, anesthesia examination, client information at the time of diagnosis, etc.) are organized via ambulant treatment, it saves bed capacity, reduces costs, and is welcomed by patients as well because they may go home a day earlier. There is no compromise on the medical preparation security. Only the process organization itself is being altered.

E.g.: While treatment and using a consistent low-pressure resection, a suprapubic catheter (SPC) generates multiple benefits: The low-pressure resection reduces the risks of the method immanent medical procedures. The SPC may then be used as a tool for efficient rinsing after the surgery. After the removal of the transurethral catheter which is usually no longer needed right after the first day of surgery, the residual urine may be controlled via the SPC. The success of the operation becomes therefore directly visible. In case the micturition is without any residual urine, typically after one day, the SPC may also be removed and patient discharge ensues. This run of events is without any problems in more than 80 % of the cases.

The whole process has cost nearly three days of hospital stay only, which is even less than DRG calculations. The cost advantage is evident. Medically, no compromises have been taken and the patient is satisfied.

Many diagnostic and treatment procedures can be checked and optimized alike.

11.4 Machinery FMEA

This is a process that mainly affects the medical device manufacturers. In clinics, this process hardly occurs. But when planning a new operating room especially with a lot of integrated technology, it is helpful to achieve proper functioning.

Here, it is useful to list the main medical purposes of the room – to plan every step and possibility in order to detect and address possible problems. In this context, the question arises: what problems may occur that you have worked out as systemically important or as secondary, for example, in a brainstorming process with all possible stakeholders from all disciplines (i.e., including building services, equipment supplier, administration, trade control if applicable, and regulators)? There are indicators for evaluation purposes, but they need to be developed for each process individually – nevertheless, its principle remains always the same.

Separately from that, data from the CIRS may also provide information on such critical processes that need to be taken into account (see Chap. 9). The processing of such problem areas can then, e.g., follow the rules of the FMEA.

11.5 Ratio Calculation

A subsequent discussion about what error to eliminate first is unavoidable if a team from different areas of a company and from different professional groups studies a process on its error proneness and causes. Errors from CIRS results and customer/patient complaints are to be given priority. A measuring unit helps in prioritizing errors found in the normal FMEA flow. That unit is called risk priority number (RPN).

11.5.1 Calculation of the Risk Priority Number (RPN)

$$RPN = B \times A \times E$$

Letters:

- B: meaning/importance of an error
- A: occurrence probability
- E: detection probability

The following values 1–10 will be assigned:

- B: very high risk: 10 points, no danger: 1 point
- A: permanent error: 10 points, unlikely occurrence of the error: 1 point
- E: very low probability of detection: 10 points, maximum detection probability: 1 point

An RPN may be calculated for each of the abovementioned FMEA groups. The higher the score, the more urgent is the elimination of the possibility of the error.

It may also be noted that the B-value is more important than, e.g., the E-value. The RPN must therefore not be used schematically but with expertise.

Thomas Schmitz-Rixen and Michael Keese

Abstract

When everything is ready to start an operation, or when there is a critical situation intraoperatively, TTO can calm down the situation, will brief everybody, and thus will lead to a smoother procedure with reduced risk.

Hospital and operating room processes are complex, and procedural mistakes can be fatal to patients. Discussing ways to prevent mistakes in this vulnerable area is becoming increasingly acceptable. The more complex and interdisciplinary a procedure, the more likely is an "adverse event" and the greater the team leader's responsibility to prevent these injurious incidents. Most serious adverse events involve wrong side or wrong site, wrong patient, or wrong procedure. A patient in Hessen suffering from bronchial carcinoma suffered an even crueler fate when the lung on the healthy side was removed instead of the lung on the diseased side. Mix-ups repeatedly occur with limb amputations (Seiden & Barach 2006), and fatal consequences of mismatched blood transfusion also occur. Devastating errors occur in operative departments with an estimated incidence of approximately 1 in 100,000 operative treatments (Rogers et al. 2006; Kwaan et al. 2006). This amounts to 5–10 major operative errors per day in the USA (Seiden & Barach 2006) and a similar incidence can be expected in Germany.

Treatment errors, such as wrong side or wrong patient, are often system errors whereby communication deficits, high workload, or time pressure play a role. Lack of medical expertise is generally not causal. Various measures have been proposed to reduce the incidence of mistakes occurring in hospitals and increasing patient safety (Ali et al. 2011; Ahmed et al. 2013; Bruce et al. 2001a, b; Rateau et al. 2011), with the aim of increasing the quality of communication between all parties involved, before and especially after a mistake has taken place. However, mistake analysis is not systematically implemented in many hospitals (Table 12.1).

Before airplane pilots begin passenger flights, they work through mandated checklists. Similar

T. Schmitz-Rixen, MD, PhD (✉)
Klinik für Gefäß- und Endovascularchirurgie und Universitären, Wundzentrum der Goethe-Universität, Chefarzt der Gefäßchirurgie am Hospital zum, Heiligen Geist gGmbH Frankfurt,
Theodor-Stern-Kai 7, Frankfurt 60590, Germany
e-mail: schmitz-rixen@em.uni-frankfurt.de

M. Keese, MD
Klinik für Gefäßchirurgie und Endovascularchirurgie, Klinikum der Goethe-Universität,
Theodor-Stern-Kai 7, Frankfurt 60590, Germany

© Springer-Verlag Berlin Heidelberg 2016
W. Merkle (ed.), *Risk Management in Medicine*, DOI 10.1007/978-3-662-47407-5_12

Table 12.1 Measures designed to increase patient safety

Measure	Description
Briefing prior to checklist application	Before first operation, consultation on all operative procedures scheduled for the day, with review of indicated treatment
M&M (morbidity and mortality) conference	Internal discussion about possible errors in patient treatment. The goal is to discuss complications and/or procedural changes to avoid repetition of treatment error
SOP (standard operating procedure)	Work instructions enabling person to carry out a procedure. Preparing and introducing a SOP include documentation, review by a second person, informing and educating the parties involved, and revision management
Clinical pathways	Instructions for standardized periprocedural course of action for itemized procedures. Useful for uncomplicated implementation of interdisciplinary and/or interprofessional procedures
Audit	Analytic method to evaluate requirements and guidelines, often in the form of quality management Audits should be carried out by qualified external personnel
Adverse events management	Constructive handling of mistakes and organizational deficits is a central element of quality management Purposeful response to mistakes and organizational deficits reduces the likelihood of repetition
Anonymous mistake reporting	Anonymous reporting of mistakes to higher-level management can prevent disciplinary or legal consequences. This type of system can be implemented externally, for example, through a medical association, or internally

checklists can increase patient safety in operating rooms and avert catastrophic complications associated with false procedures on false patients. For this reason surgeons have long been scrutinizing safety procedures utilized in aviation. Not only are technical aspects covered in aviation checklists; another aim is to curtail human failure due to lack of communication and rigid hierarchy. A worldwide WHO campaign called "Safe Surgery Saves Lives" is transferring aviation principles to the operating room (http://www.who.int/patientsafety/safesurgery/en/). Since June 2008, a 19-point perioperative checklist in modified form has been introduced into German clinics (Figs. 12.1 and 12.2).

Checklists may differ according to individual hospital specifications. However, the checklist should be uniform within the hospital to avoid misunderstandings during interdisciplinary procedures. According to WHO standards, the checklists are divided into three main sections. Aside from preoperative measures carried out by the nursing staff and ward physician a "Sign-In" should occur directly before the patient enters the operating room. Patient identity and the marked side should be compared with the signed,

informed consent form. Any discrepancy requires the surgeon's personal appearance to clarify the situation according to patient records or by ordering reassessment. Not till then may the patient be admitted to the operating room. A perioperative "Team-Time-Out" then follows with all persons present taking part in the operation (surgeons, anesthetists, and nursing staff). Since the providing surgeon at this point is standing sterile at the operating table, it is recommended that the Team-Time-Out checklist be systematically read aloud by a member of the nursing staff.

Involving the nursing staff strengthens team spirit, making each person in the operating room aware of his/her responsibility for the patient's safety, regardless of position in the hierarchy. Verbal confirmation of patient identity, body side, procedure, and goal of the operation follows. Critical operative steps or anticipated difficulties in anesthesia management should be pointed out. The anesthetist must remind the surgeon of risks, which could influence intraoperative decisions. The nursing staff confirms instrument sterility and the availability of correct implants and special requirements or equipment.

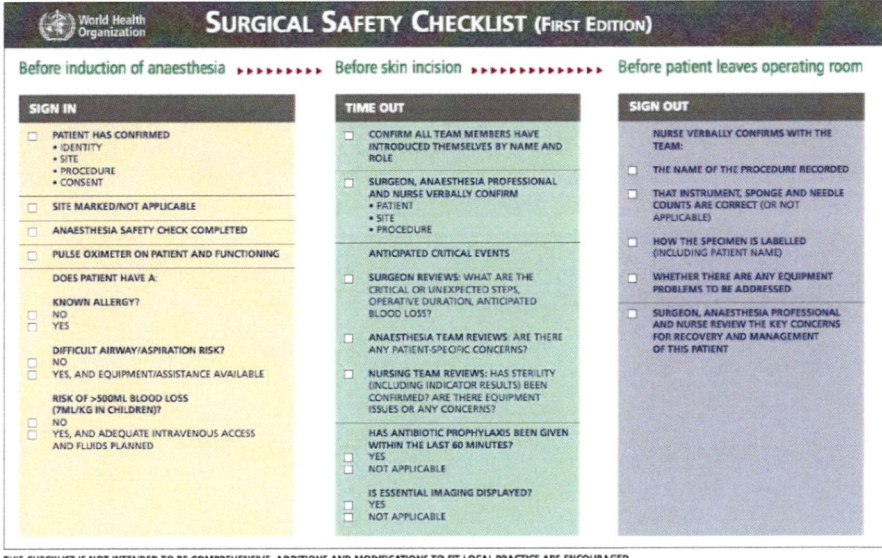

Fig. 12.1 WHO's "Team-Time-Out" checklist (http://www.who.int/patientsafety/safesurgery/ss_checklist/en/)

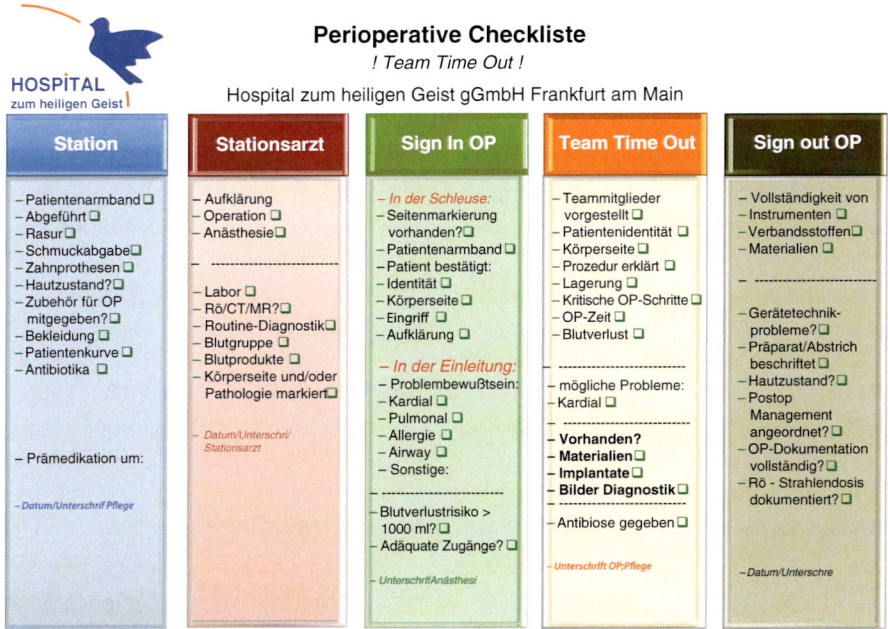

Fig. 12.2 "Team-Time-Out" checklist in the "Hospital zum heiligen Geist gGmbH," Frankfurt am Main, Germany

The availability of implants should be affirmed by the ward physician or providing surgeon on the day prior to the surgical procedure. Simple measures such as a "Time Out" sign over the scalpel on the instrument table can help maintain a standardized Team-Time-Out procedure (Fig. 12.3). This can also take place during the current operation itself in case unclear points might occur suddenly, e.g., unclear mass, individual anatomical condition, etc.

In postoperative "Sign-Out," the surgical nursing staff verbally confirms completeness of

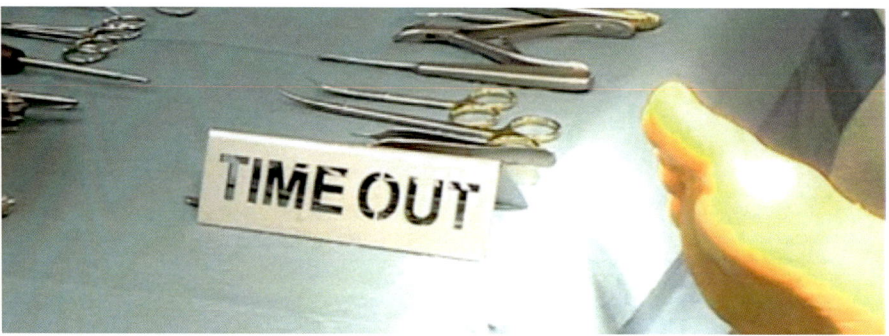

Fig. 12.3 Time Out sign lying over the scalpel until Team-Time-Out is completed

instruments and surgical textiles. Postoperative care is detailed by the surgeon and anesthetist. Problems encountered with medical equipment are documented to implement timely replacement. Time expended for working through each of the three checklists is maximally 2 min, which is less than the combined time spent for delays in procedure generally caused by urgent telephone calls into the operating room.

Within the framework of an international, multicenter study, it was convincingly demonstrated in 2009 that the introduction of the WHO Surgical Safety Checklist into operating rooms led to a significant decrease in postoperative mortality and complications (Haynes et al. 2009). Inclusion of 8 hospitals, spread over the world (Toronto, Canada; New Delhi, India; Amman, Jordan; Auckland, New Zealand; Manila, Philippines; Ifakara, Tanzania; London, England; and Seattle, WA. USA) ensured a diverse socio-economic background for the investigation. The study covered a prospective analysis of clinical procedures and outcome in 3733 patients (older than 16 years, excluding cardiac surgery). Directly thereafter, upon introducing the checklists, the complication rate and outcome of a further 3955 surgical patients were catalogued. Endpoints of the study were complications and 30-day perioperative mortality, associated with the surgical procedure. A significant decrease in mortality from 1.5 to 0.8 % was achieved after introducing the WHO checklists. The complication rate after introduction of the checklists was also significantly decreased from 11 to 7 % (Haynes et al. 2011). These improvements did

not depend upon public service obligation or hospital location. Since all of the hospitals already had surgical safety policies in place, the significance of introducing these particular checklists is obvious. Checklists increase patient safety (Lingard et al. 2008; Makary et al. 2006; Sexton et al. 2006), but noncompliance hinders their undeniable benefit. The more complicated checklists are, the less they are employed (Poon et al. 2013). But compliance varies even with the standard straightforward WHO checklists. Retrospective analysis shows that inclusion of the surgical nursing staff and checking the availability of implants and essential imaging are the checklist points most often neglected. Generally, during Team-Time-Out, surgeon and anesthetist dominance has been noted and criticized (Rydenfalt et al. 2013). By ensuring that the unsterile colleague from the nursing staff ("Springer") works through the Team-Time-Out checklist point by point, not only does the nursing staff become actively involved, but compliance of all other team members is increased.

Quality management (QM) can ensure that Team-Time-Out checklists are implemented. In the Johann Wolfgang Goethe University Hospital, Frankfurt am Main, audits are carried out every 3 months to check the compliance of the operating room team members in completing checklists. QM's first step is to check whether the checklists are in the patient files.

Hundred percent compliance is hardly possible due to emergency procedures carried out during the night. Figure 12.4 shows a compliance analysis of checklist completeness for team

Checklisten - Gefäßchirurgie

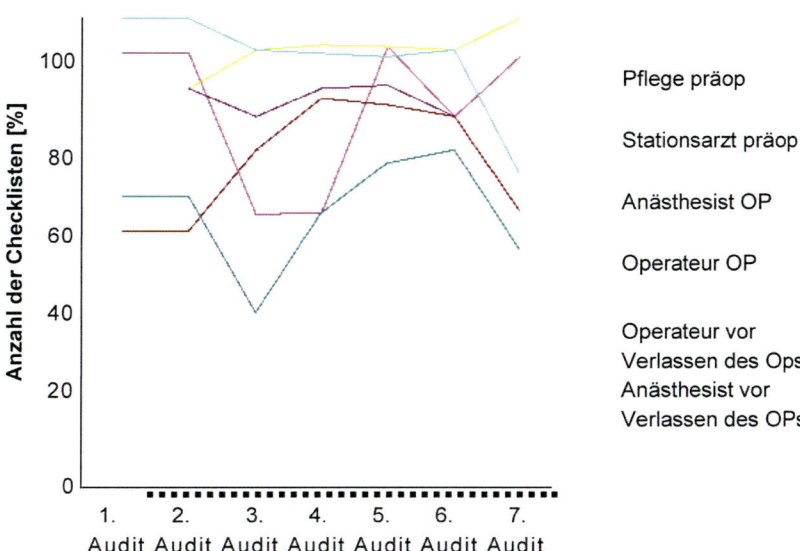

Fig. 12.4 Compliance of team members in filling out Team-Time-Out checklists for all operations in the Department of Vascular and Endovascular Surgery at the Goethe University hospital

members in the Department of Vascular and Endovascular Surgery.

According to Poon et al. (2013), compliance, upon which the Team-Time-Out checklist rests, lies between 50 and 80 % for different members of the operating team. The compilation from the Department of Vascular and Endovascular Surgery, shown above, shows that preoperatively, relatively high compliance is found for the nursing crew, ward physician, and anesthetist. Unfortunately, internal auditing did not increase compliance. In an effort to increase compliance, a detailed, personalized analysis will follow. This is of central importance since it has been proven that strict implementation of checklists in every surgical field leads to a decrease in postoperative morbidity and mortality. An alternative to improving checklist compliance is to introduce external audits. This method has been shown to be more effective than internal audits or educational measures (Flodgren et al. 2011).

To err is human and operating rooms, populated by humans, are places where mistakes occur. More important than sanctions directed against individuals who neglect checklists is to

increase awareness about how important the checklists are. Concentrating on important procedural steps by using the checklists sharpens the view of the procedure as a whole and intensifies the awareness of responsibility in bringing the patient safely and effectively through the operation. Therefore, it is imperative to introduce measures to make operative procedures less susceptible to mistakes.

Conclusion

To significantly reduce perioperative mortality and morbidity, the nationwide introduction of Team-Time-Out checklists is necessary and should be an integral element of any operational quality management program. All facilities offering operative and interventional procedures can profit from Team-Time-Out. It is crucial to motivate all team members and to maintain motivation. Certainly, introducing Team-Time-Out requires some effort, and department heads must serve as role models. However, once successfully installed into the operational procedure, routine Team-Time-Out costs little time-wise, actually saves time in the long run, improves team spirit as a positive side effect, and, most importantly, morbidity and mortality are reduced.

Acknowledgement The authors acknowledge the language expertise of Mrs. Karen Nelson

Literature

Ahmed A, Sadadcharam G, Andrews E (2013) The road map to better knowledge? Care pathways as an educational tool during surgical internship. J Surg Educ 70:273–278

Ali M, Osborne A, Bethune R, Pullyblank A (2011) Preoperative surgical briefings do not delay operating room start times and are popular with surgical team members. J Patient Saf 7:139–143

Bruce J, Russell EM, Mollison J, Krukowski ZH (2001a) The quality of measurement of surgical wound infection as the basis for monitoring: a systematic review. J Hosp Infect 49:99–108

Bruce J, Russell EM, Mollison J, Krukowski ZH (2001b) The measurement and monitoring of surgical adverse events. Health Technol Assess 5:1–194

Flodgren G, Pomey MP, Taber SA, Eccles MP (2011) Effectiveness of external inspection of compliance with standards in improving healthcare organisation behaviour, healthcare professional behaviour or patient outcomes. Cochrane Database Syst Rev (11):CD008992

Haynes AB, Weiser TG, Berry WR et al (2009) A surgical safety checklist to reduce morbidity and mortality in a global population. N Engl J Med 360:491–499

Haynes AB, Weiser TG, Berry WR et al (2011) Changes in safety attitude and relationship to decreased postoperative morbidity and mortality following implementation of a checklist-based surgical safety intervention. BMJ Qual Saf 20:102–107

Kwaan MR, Studdert DM, Zinner MJ, Gawande AA (2006) Incidence, patterns, and prevention of wrong-site surgery. Arch Surg 141:353–357; discussion 7–8

Lingard L, Regehr G, Orser B et al (2008) Evaluation of a preoperative checklist and team briefing among surgeons, nurses, and anesthesiologists to reduce failures in communication. Arch Surg 143:12–17; discussion 8

Makary MA, Sexton JB, Freischlag JA et al (2006) Operating room teamwork among physicians and nurses: teamwork in the eye of the beholder. J Am Coll Surg 202:746–752

Poon SJ, Zuckerman SL, Mainthia R et al (2013) Methodology and bias in assessing compliance with a surgical safety checklist. Jt Comm J Qual Patient Saf 39:77–82

Rateau F, Levraut L, Colombel AL et al (2011) Check-list "Patient Safety" in the operating room: one year experience of 40,000 surgical procedures at the university hospital of Nice. Ann Fr Anesth Reanim 30:479–483

Rogers SO Jr, Gawande AA, Kwaan M et al (2006) Analysis of surgical errors in closed malpractice claims at 4 liability insurers. Surgery 140:25–33

Rydenfalt C, Johansson G, Odenrick P, Akerman K, Larsson PA (2013) Compliance with the WHO Surgical Safety Checklist: deviations and possible improvements. Int J Qual Health Care 25:182–187

Seiden SC, Barach P (2006) Wrong-side/wrong-site, wrong-procedure, and wrong-patient adverse events: are they preventable? Arch Surg 141:931–939

Sexton JB, Makary MA, Tersigni AR et al (2006) Teamwork in the operating room: frontline perspectives among hospitals and operating room personnel. Anesthesiology 105:877–884

Nina Walter

Abstract

Formalistic check of failures is – no doubt – helpful in order to avoid them.

Medicine processes are very complex; thus simple check procedures cannot be successful at last. Peer review uses experts to look after team behavior, complex procedures, process management, etc. because they are able to understand even non-formalistic processes and can judge them as correct or incorrect.

Details are pointed out.

The process of identifying and minimizing risks makes one thing apparent.

As Johann Wolfgang von Goethe, the great German poet, correctly pointed out: "Man errs, till he has ceased to strive."

Not only poets and philosophers have come to this conclusion. Current research and numerous scientific studies have clearly shown time and time again that human beings as an acting entity are a crucial, essential or decisive risk factor in any process.

To minimize these risks, different approaches and procedures that mutually enrich and reinforce each other are being used.

The most relevant ones are compiled in this textbook.

But an unrecognized small blind spot may remain, even if the person involved acts to the best of his/her knowledge and beliefs, processes checklists continuously, and critically scrutinizes all actions.

This is where the peer review procedure comes into play in: an unbureaucratic, flexible procedure focusing on collegial exchange as an instrument of improving quality measures.

13.1 Definition

Attempting to find a definition for "peer review," one comes up with answers related to the assessment of scientific output, specifically publications. A key characteristic is the assessment by peers from the same specialization.

More detailed and focusing on patient care, "quality management in medicine" defines peer review as an "ongoing systematical and critical reflection by several individuals aiming for

N. Walter, MA
St. Leiterin Stabsstelle Qualitätssicherung,
Versorgungsmanagement und Gesundheitsökonomie,
Landesärztekammer Hessen,
Im Vogelsgesang 3, Frankfurt 60488, Germany
e-mail: nina.walter@laekh.de

© Springer-Verlag Berlin Heidelberg 2016
W. Merkle (ed.), *Risk Management in Medicine*, DOI 10.1007/978-3-662-47407-5_13

continuous improvement of the quality of patient care through usage of a structured process assessing the efficiency of themselves, and others, within their occupational group."

The peer review procedure encourages exchange of knowledge, information, and experience in a structured professional environment.

A clear indication that the medical profession has chosen the right path implementing peer review procedures is the fact that the main focus coincides with the three fundamental objectives defined by the German Association for Evaluation: professionalization of evaluation, integration of differing perspectives, and promotion of information flow and dialogue.

13.2 History

The Royal Society of England, as well as many other scientific societies founded in the seventeenth century repeatedly saw the reliability of their scientific findings and experiments questioned. Most authors regard these times as the initial progress of peer review methods. Members of such societies were generally classified as trustworthy, and their work was recognized and in principle acknowledged.

Members of societies often vouched for the works of external or lower-ranking scientists and the quality of their respective work. Frequently, such experiments had to be repeated in the presence of members to be verified.

The beginnings of structured peer review procedures dates back to the 1750s, when Henry Oldenburg, editor of "Philosophical Transactions" founded in 1655 in London, was faced with a dilemma: as a theologian, he considered himself unqualified to appropriately assess the quality of submitted essays on scientific topics. He therefore delegated the task to other scientists who were known to be competent or experienced in on those subjects. This method was adapted by other scientific publications and has since become an established procedure.

The use of this method for clinical treatment processes and the direct evaluation of patient care was not introduced until much later, approximately at the beginning of the twentieth century. In the 1970s, several medical societies in the USA defined their views on the integration of "medical audits" or peer reviews for quality improvement.

The decisive impetus for the establishment of the procedure in Germany was given by the "Initiative for Quality Medicine," the "German Society for Anesthesiology and Intensive Care Medicine," the "German Interdisciplinary Association for Emergency and Intensive Care Medicine," and the "Alliance of German Anesthesiologists."

To implement the peer review procedure across the broad, the German Medical Association created the curriculum "Medical Peer Review," issued in 2011. It provides an overview of the theoretical background, and its chapter "Qualification Concept" details the range of expertise a peer should possess and how this range can be achieved using the modules presented as part of the curriculum. The comprehensive curriculum can be accessed on the website of the German Medical Association.

(Bundesärztekammer): (http://www.bundesaerztekammer.de/downloads/Curriculum_Aerztliches_Peer_Review1.pdf)

13.3 Curriculum of the German Medical Association

The improvement of the quality of medical work is one of the basic needs of physicians. Colleagues are determined to remain in full control of their actions at all times. The bureaucratic measurements required are often disproportionate to the tangible benefits when the legal quality control measures are applied.

As a voluntary procedure of physicians provided to their peers, the peer review procedure constitutes a deliberate countertype.

The curriculum presents the range of competences of a peer clearly displayed in tabular form. This compilation forms the core of the whole curriculum and describes the prerequisites for an effective risk management in general (Table 13.1).

Table 13.1 Competency profile of peers

Competence category	A good peer
Knowledge	Has long-term professional expert knowledge and experience in the quality areas to be evaluated Has been active in a leading function in clinic/practice Has experience in the areas of quality assurance and promoting quality Knows the current models of quality management and the principles of evaluation Is aware of objective, subject-matter, process, and versions of peer reviews Knows the roles and tasks of the peers involved
Skills	Is able to analyze in a patient-oriented way Applies the basic principles of organizational development Is able to collect, analyze, and evaluate qualitative data Adheres to the rules of the respective peer review procedure
Social competence	Cooperates with the members of the peer review team Uses appropriate discussion techniques such as solution-based dialogue in an advisory capacity Actively requests other points of view Shows respect for differing points of view Gives short, precise, and intelligible oral and written accounts of his evaluation Appropriately notes criticism and voices criticism Handles conflicts in a solution-oriented matter
Self-competence	Reflects on potential conflicts of interest with constructive consequences Personifies the peer as an empathetic "critical friend" and peer advisor Reflects on lessons learned from his own experiences and those of others Focuses on potential solutions (versus problems) Works meticulously Acts fair and responsible

The concept for qualification is based on the so-called Competency Model of the Initiative of the German Qualification Requirements for Lifelong Learning (DQR). It aims at preparing participants for the independent adaptation of peer review procedures by providing theoretical and practical learning modules.

The sequence of the modules replicates the phases of a peer review procedure and is taught in a 1.5–2-day seminar. Peer qualification is completed with two practical reviews which have to be conducted in the presence of experienced peers.

At the the basic/fundamental issues of the peer review are the dialogue, the personal examination/observation (onsite), and the exchange of views on the matters perceived.

Since peers are required to give critical feedback during this process, the training concept emphasizes the aspects of dialogue, self-competence, and social competence. A defined objective is the command of the basic principles of solution-oriented communication (see Table 13.2).

The treatment process does not just involve physicians but other professional groups as well. This means that all parties involved need to be integrated in a combined effort for quality improvement and risk management. Only an interdisciplinary and cross-occupational approach can offer comprehensive and sustainable solutions.

The German Medical Association has, under its jurisdiction, developed the curriculum "Medical Peer Review" but continues to emphasize that it can and should be used for multiprofessional education seminars.

13.4 Peer Review Procedure

A peer review consists of three phases (see Fig. 13.1):

1. Self-assessment
2. External assessment and exchange between colleagues and interaction in the context of a peer collaboration
3. Reporting

Table 13.2 Modules of qualification concepts of the curriculum "Medical Peer Review" of the German Medical Association

Module	Form of mediation	Phase	Teaching units (unit = 45 min)
1. Peer reviews in the context of quality management and evaluation, strategy/methods used	Theory (training)	Background knowledge	3 units
2. Tasks and role/position of peer	Theory/training	Phases 1–3	2 units
3. Data collection, data analysis, and evaluation	Theory/training preparation	Phase 2	3 units
4. Design and planning of a peer review	Theory/training preparation	Phase 1	2 units
5. Feedback and reports	Theory/training	Phases 2–3	2 units
6. Personal competency Self management Solution-oriented dialogue Handling of conflicts, criticism, resistance	Training	Phases 1–3	Cross-section module 180 min (4 units)
Two practice reviews	Practical application (trial participation in two peer reviews alongside an experienced peer)		16 units

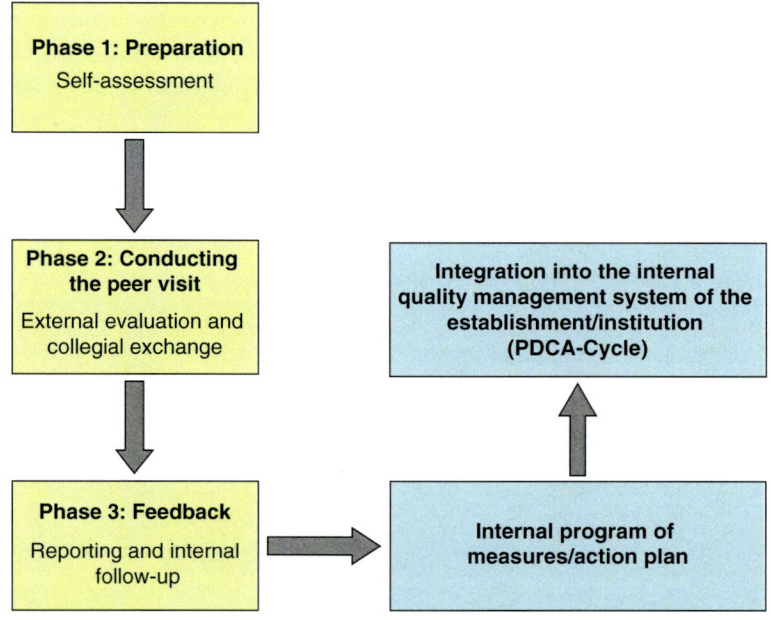

Fig. 13.1 The passway of peer review

It is followed by a subsequent internal follow-up procedure, in which an action plan is developed.

The self-assessment is conducted by the unit to be visited and reviewed.

The corresponding evaluation scheme is a standardized/structured survey. In intensive care medicine, the survey consists of 60 questions which are divided into the sections: structural quality, process quality, and performance quality. Since the procedure is applicable in any field of work, the surveys are selected according a specialization as well as to specific agreements.

The results are given to the peers before or during the peer visit.

The survey providing the guideline for the peer review in intensive care medicine was developed by the German Society for Anesthesiology and Intensive Care Medicine and by the German Interdisciplinary Association for Intensive and Emergency Care (DIVI). Comprehensive questionnaires based on clinically approved certification procedures and qualitative indicators of intensive care medicine served as a base for the survey design.

The "Initiative Quality Medicine" has integrated peer reviews into their QM and conducted 67 peer review procedures between 2009 and 2011.

The daylong visit by the peer team includes an introductory discussion and an onsite viewing of aspects and areas specified in the questionnaire, reviewing of files, and appraising of processes. The peer team then conducts an external assessment, referring to the previously submitted self-assessment.

In the form of a cooperative exchange, the reviewed department receives an oral feedback that serves as a basis for potential improvements and respective measures of implementation.

Achievable targets and strategic improvement measures with clear time limits are proposed after a concluding discussion with management, administration, medical director, and patient care management.

The final written report is submitted to the institution shortly thereafter and provides additional important notes and recommendations of action, if possible in the form of a SWOT analysis (analysis of strengths, weaknesses, opportunities, threats) according to the results of the peer reviews.

Subsequently, it is the responsibility of the institution evaluated to establish a road map to achieve continuous improvement to be integrated into their quality management plan.

13.5   Evaluation of the Evaluation

Between 2010 and 2012, the seminar "Peer Review" based on the curriculum of the German Medical Association has been attended by more than 300 participants.

Thirty-six peer reviews have been conducted in intensive care units as well as in units for Transfusion Medicine.

The first 17 courses held in the regional associations Baden-Württemberg, Hamburg, Berlin, and Schleswig-Holstein were evaluated based on structured questionnaires.

The objective of the collection of data was to determine how the participants rated the course and its practical relevance as well as which of the topics covered were of importance to them. First results showed that participants' rating of the seminar were predominantly positive.

It should be noted that the participants consisted mainly of chief and senior physicians, who rated both content and form of the qualification measures as beneficial and deemed the practical application onsite as a conductive instrument for quality development.

To be provided with an essential tool for quality assurance and improvement that could be used and continuously developed through exchange with colleagues was important to many participants and was praised as an innovation.

The president of the regional medical association of Berlin has therefore characterized the peer review procedure as an "inherent traditional medical care procedure."

13.6 Conclusion and Long-Term Vision/Future Prospects

The implementation of the curriculum "Medical Peer Review" and the corresponding feedback lead to the conclusion that the contents and didactic advice were effectively and positively received.

Due to the positive response, the German Medical Association has decided to actively support a nationwide expansion of "peer reviews" and has established a working group to develop a "Guideline for Peer Reviews" (http://www.bundesaerztekammer.de/fileadmin/user_upload/downloads/Leitfaden_Aerztliches-Peer-Review_2014.pdf).

So far the procedure is mainly being applied in the areas of intensive care medicine and hemotherapy. But word spread about the positive user experience and professionals of other fields and specialization have expressed their interest to utilize the procedure for their purposes.

Further expansion of the procedure would be desirable – it supports physicians and multi-professional teams in their collegial interaction to integrate quality and risk management into their day-to-day clinical work while keeping bureaucracy at a minimum.

During the preparation phase, a look at the methods of the FMEA proves beneficial for identifying and prioritizing the problem areas to be assessed.

Cord-H. Becker and Walter Merkle

Quality and safety are of primary importance. This is why it is essential to form a working team based upon trust (cf. Chaps. 1 and 6). The members of this team must be able to function when meeting for the first time, even if they are not acquainted with or close to one another.

While most chapters of this book focused on error theory and individual error risk, CRM describes an error prevention theory. Cooperation with others is often centered on problem solving. Since errors are bound to occur when people work together, this cooperation must be "organized."

After several air crashes, some of them quite spectacular, NASA attempted to get to the roots of this high number of accidents in a workshop held in 1979. The results were clear about one thing – human error was the predominant cause of those investigated accidents. There were deficits in communication as well as conflicts over authority within the crew. Furthermore, procedures were ignored or operations in the cockpit were disregarded, resulting in a complex interplay of chains of mistakes, known generally in its simplified form as pilot error Cooper et al. (1980).

This start-up resulted in airlines as well as other high-risk industries (e.g., nuclear energy, aerospace, chemical plants) developing measures which led to CRM. By now, CRM is not only found at all American and European airlines but has become a requirement for pilots and other crew members worldwide.

A prime example of the success of CRM is the famous ditching of US Airways flight 1549 on the Hudson River. Despite a catastrophic technical failure, the crew succeeded in saving all passengers' lives. In the final analysis, this happened through teamwork and a rescue strategy developed instantaneously by Captain Sullenberger, who was flying the plane; instruments on the copilot's side also ceased functioning due to engine failure National Transportation Safety Board (2009).

In contrast, there has previously been no applied CRM in the field of medicine with few exceptions (albeit especially in the field of surgery, other invasive procedures, or even medication where the risk for diagnostic errors (malpractice) is evident, conclusive frameworks do exist to deal with these errors).

The Gynecological Clinic of the University of Vienna has established a department devoted solely to risk management and patient safety.

Insights gained from the industrial sectors in which error management lead to risk management, in other words in the high-risk sectors, can also be applied to the medical field – problems

C.-H. Becker (✉)
ATS Aviation Training Support,
Gustav-Freytag-Str. 15, Wiesbaden 65189, Germany
e-mail: cord@cordbecker.de

W. Merkle, MD
Riskmanager in Medicine Specialist in Urology,
Management Expert for Hospitals (VWA),
German Diagnostic Clinic – Helios Clinic,
Aukammallee 33, Wiesbaden D 65191, Germany
e-mail: Risikomanagement.Merkle@hotmail.de

© Springer-Verlag Berlin Heidelberg 2016
W. Merkle (ed.), *Risk Management in Medicine*, DOI 10.1007/978-3-662-47407-5_14

are more or less of the same nature, namely, human.

Error Recognition

- Heeding human factors and performance limits
- Dealing with working errors, organizational culture
- Teamwork

These are the key issues for the successful implementation of strategies of safety.

It is important to identify potential errors (see Chap. 11). Near-mistakes in which "everything turned out okay after all" are to be analyzed (compare Chap. 9). Effects of errors are to be minimized as it is an irrefutable fact that people make mistakes.

One for all and all for one !
This saying of the famous Three Musketeers from the novel by A. Dumas sums up the essence of teamwork.

The Swiss cheese model (see Chap. 4) explains how this working together can result in successful error prevention.

If the chain of errors is not broken by someone in the team, complications in dealing with it arise. The results are human suffering and legal consequences (compare Chap. 15).

Team building is easier said than done. When a team is formed, including teams formed in a hospital setting, it seldom consists of a group of personal friends. In general, it is an element such as a working schedule which results in an arbitrary number of people coming together to complete a given task, in other words, coming together to form a team, for example, an OP team. Especially in large clinics it is common for people who hardly know each other to work together. That notwithstanding, the goal is the precise, optimal, flawless treatment of a patient.

Out of a randomly chosen group of employees, a team must form which can, if needed, "ditch a plane onto the Hudson River." How does the field of aviation organize this?

The solution is CRM.

Personal interests must be subjugated to team goals. How Captain Sullenberger achieved this

until landing his aircraft on the Hudson was told in an interview:

The interview shows what enormous time pressure the crew was under. In training, these emergency scenarios (even if not under these exact extreme circumstances) allow for the crew to develop and practice a framework for an emergency. Captain Sullenberger said in his interview, "… I had to force myself to use my training." The division of duties in the cockpit shows how precisely the crew followed the "golden rules" of the aircraft manufacturer Airbus Industries: respect task sharing. (Captain Sullenberger takes over the controls and communication with air traffic control while the copilot goes through the electronic and evacuation checklist). Belonging to this is the "rule" – own responsibility (of task) while keeping the other (crew member) in loop.

When speaking of the Hudson River landing, no pilot will speak of heroism, least of all Captain Sullenberger. This was an outstandingly professional achievement with Captain Sullenberger in command. This accomplishment did not stop with the landing. Captain Sullenberger's last statement in the interview is "… and I had a job to do." What he meant was rescuing the passengers – a responsibility of the captain, provided that he is able to do so.

Starting with its inception in 1979, there have been five different developmental stages for CRM.

The first phase began in 1981 with United Airlines. The focus was on psychological factors. Training centered on dismissing hierarchical relationships while offering mutual support, meaning the copilot was encouraged to point out the captain's mistakes, so that the captain had a chance to recognize and correct them in time. That presupposed that the captain encouraged his team to address mistakes or inaccuracies irrespective of person or position (compare Chaps. 1 and 6). This CRM was exclusively for cockpit members, *Cockpit* Resource Management.

In the second phase, the cabin crew would become involved in this *crew* resource management. Briefing and stress management on board were the topics of this training. Breaking the chain of errors before an accident occurred was also taught.

It was only in the third phase that technical trainings specific for flying were added to these psychological approaches.

Additionally programs were added to examine so-called human skills which were not directly related to operating the aircraft (compare Chap. 3).

CRM became institutionalized in the fourth phase, becoming an integral part of basic and advanced flight training. This is still the case today.

The concept of active error management was developed out of the fifth phase of CRM. Precisely because so many people of different nationalities work together in the field of aviation, there are many different frames of reference for dealing with errors Helmreich et al. (1999). These multicultural teams, arising from present-day patterns of migration, are becoming almost the rule, even in hospitals. One more reason to move away from these influences is by placing the focus on team building; leaving it to chance then renders it susceptible to errors. One need not even consider differences in ethnic groups to understand the difficulties in forming teams. Variations in early childhood development due to diverse social background and home life, peer group norms during puberty – all of these lead to complicating the task of team building. It is not enough to just mandate a team; it has to function. Only then is a team not just a "mixed-up bunch of people."

This is how teams in aviation train on one hand optimized human interaction and on the other hand active error management within the context of CRM. The influence of psychology on CRM's beginning stages hasn't been mitigated, but instead is always present.

The goal of the CRM process is first error prevention by the team itself (!), as every individual makes mistakes. Further, mistakes should be discovered before they lead to a fatal crash. Finally, mistakes should be analyzed for learning experiences due to the very reason that they have occurred (compare book on complications in urology).

CRM as a specific team training can be seen in many videos in the web. Two things are practiced - first, preventing errors which arise from human shortcomings; second, transparent operational procedures.

Error prevention strategies include;

- Realizing that you make mistakes
- Recognizing your performance limits
- Accepting that fatigue and stress increase error probability
- Distrusting your own abilities/your own sense of security
- Simplifying procedures and instructions
- Using checklists and guidelines[1]

Training contents of CRM include;

- Uncovering hidden resources of the team
- Undoing entrenched (problematic) behavioral patterns
- Learning to accept criticism (objectively, not personally!)
- Developing security
- Becoming aware of and accepting human error susceptibility
- Simulating low hierarchies which allow for the flow of information
- Implementing the notion of team spirit
- Emphasizing open communication (compare OTAS)
- Training decision-making processes of the team

These measures will not reduce the high number of risks, but these risks can be more easily detected and therefore minimized.

This is why CRM is a permanent process. Continual training is necessary to counteract human forgetfulness and complacency.

A clinic which adopts and actualizes these CRM procedures raises employee motivation and reduces the rate of errors, a benefit for patients and the clinic alike. In times of tense economic conditions, this should not be disregarded too quickly.

A more beneficial win-win situation is hard to imagine.

---

[1] Cave –Guidelines in the field of medicine are not directives (compare Chaps. 1, 6 and 15).

References

Cooper GE, White MD, Lauber JK (1980) Resource management on the flightdeck – proceedings of a NASA/industry workshop (NASA CP-2120) Meffett Field, CA: NASA Ames Research Center

Helmreich RL, Merritt AC, Sherman PJ (1997) Research project evaluates the effect of national culture on flight crew behaviour

Helmreich RL et al. (1999) The evolution of crew resource management training in commercial aviation. Int J Aviation Psychol; 9(1), 19–32

National Transportation Safety Board (2009) Accident Report NTSB/AAR-10/03 PB2010-910403, http://www.ntsb.gov/doclib/reports/2010/AAR1003.pdf, Page 91 (abgerufen am 25.08.2013)

Stephan Krempel

Abstract

The specific German way of dealing with malpractice is highlighted.

The German Medical Liability Law had not been codified until the so-called Patient Rights Act came into effect in February 2013.

Up to that point, the treatment contract had followed the rules of service contract law (§§ 611 ff. BGB). A "new type of contract" was created with the introduction of the Patient Rights Act, the treatment contract according to § 630 a BGB, which provides for the exchange of medical services against payment. This is a "specific type of contract" that not only regulates physicians' activities but also the activities of other members of the medical profession (see Wagner, Kodifikation des Arzthaftungsrechts, VersR 2012, 790 ff). It incorporates midwives, perinatal nurses, masseurs, medical balneotherapists, psychologists, psychotherapists, ergotherapists, speech therapists, and dentists as well (see Wagner, loc. cit.).

The regulations of the Patient Rights Act are, however, no novelty; they just couch past and present court rulings summed up in legal articles (§§ 620 ff. BGB).

German physician liability law/medical malpractice law is eventually governed by the burden of proof. The law initially defines the rights and duties of the parties involved (medical professional and patient) and finally regularizes – in § 630 b BGB – the prerequisites as effective consent being the requirement to justify bodily injury/damage to person related to any physical intervention. Details ensuing from the obligation to informing the patient are regulated by § 630 e BGB, meaning the patient must be informed in detail of all major circumstances needed for his/her consent as to the kind, extent, and execution of medical action, possible sequelae, and risks linked with the procedure, its necessity and urgency, agreements, and prospects regarding diagnosis and treatment. Alternatives to the suggested procedures must clearly be pointed out when there are several medically similarly and commonly indicated methods, which may lead to significantly less stress and risks or different prognosis for cure. This also encompasses the question of "conservative versus surgical procedure," outpatient versus inpatient treatment, especially when an intervention is being suggested that is not contained in the catalog of outpatient procedures, e.g., varied types of incision or surgical techniques.

S. Krempel
Fachanwalt für Medizinrecht,
Futterstr. 3, Saarbrücken 66111, Germany
e-mail: kanzlei@anwaltskanzlei-krempel.de

© Springer-Verlag Berlin Heidelberg 2016
W. Merkle (ed.), *Risk Management in Medicine*, DOI 10.1007/978-3-662-47407-5_15

In any case, information will have to be provided in a face-to-face meeting by either the attending physician or by a knowledgeable third party with professional credentials, while documents are (merely) being referred supplementarily and which the patient needs to receive in print. This excludes simply handing over an information form – for instance, by Diomed™ or ProCompliance™ – with the verbal request to read it carefully and to sign it, even when the patient has been told that he/she is welcome to ask any questions he/she may have after reading the text.

It's, moreover, paramount that information is provided in due time so that the patient may base his informed consent on well-founded considerations. Early patient information – the more serious and hazardous the operation (diagnostic intervention) is expected to be – is the principle behind this stipulation. It's desirable to inform the patient prior to inpatient admission – and best even before an appointment for surgery has been made, leaving the patient enough time to get a second opinion if he/she so wishes. It goes without saying that patient information has to be tailored to the patient's capacity of understanding.

Lawmakers provided (§ 630 e section 3 BGB) that patient information/informed consent is exempted under particular exceptions, which would include unpostponable interventions and/or the patient's explicit refusal of information. The latter has to be approached with particular precaution: It will take scrutinized documentation and calling in of witnesses, who should sign that they had been informed thereof. This paper must be put into the patient's file and/or be added as a document in the electronic documentation.

The physician needs to furnish proof that he has informed the patient accordingly regarding the risks of intervention. He can do that by presenting his documentation supplemented by his own hearing if that documentation is sufficient. Of course, witnesses may come in in addition, when, for example, the hospital "alone" is being sued, and the informing physician is available as a witness. In nonhospital, office-based settings, nurse practitioners or doctor's receptionists may qualify to bear witness.

The development of standards is recommended in this respect since the hearing of evidence with regard to proper information often takes place years after the treatment at stake and witnesses' recollections are naturally vague; they are unable to remember patients who had come to the office 5 or even 12 years ago. In such cases, jurisdiction has clearly acknowledged that it will suffice if witnesses (can) describe a common procedure, moreover confirming that there had been no deviation from the standard.

Dispute arises over and again whether certain measures had been taken, examinations been carried out or been advised, or if the patient had been given behavioral instructions. Article (§) 630 f, section 2 BGB describes the attending physician's obligation to document in the patient file each and every medical approach and its results, which, by professional perspective, might be essential as to present and future therapy. This particularly applies to the patient's history, diagnoses, tests, examination results, findings, treatments and their effect, interventions and their outcome, informed consent, and previous information. Within this context, please mind § 630 a, section 3 BGB, which assumes that no measure had been taken if pertinent medically indicated treatment options and their results are not documented in the patient file – or if the patient file had been disposed of prior to the 10 years' safekeeping period (§ 630 f, section 3 BGB).

This assumption may, of course, be contradicted by testimonial proof; it would, however, seem quite unlikely that another physician working in that office or a nurse practitioner or other staff still has a precise recollection of what had been done a decade ago, an ultrasound examination, for instance, without a printout at hand or any other documentation in this regard.

The author is convinced that erroneous or negligent documentation really figures large in the processing of medical malpractice warrants of attorney. In fact, it often happens and not just rarely that experts will deny malpractice, whereas patients maintain that they had not been duly informed of the risks of the intervention or not been alerted to alternative treatments, and at loss is the physician who fails to furnish satisfactory evidence for lack of a diligent documentation in terms of indisputable informed consent. If it is merely a question of therapeutic information or medical safety advisory (i.e., information on all circumstances which should be observed to ascertain a curative outcome, compliance to treatment, and the avoidance of possible self-endangerment), the onus of proof is cast upon patient; he/she has to produce evidence that the physician neglected his duties to the effect of injuriousness to the patient's health. Since medical safety advisory – in jurisdiction – may lead to petty, simple malpractice, the burden of proof rests with the patient.

In the event of so-called grave malpractice, however, the burden of proof is shifted to the physician; the assumption behind it is that injuriousness to health was caused by malpractice. The same holds true when the attending physician, by passive negligence or nonfeasance, failed to make or corroborate a medically indicated diagnosis early enough, inasmuch as this finding would have most probably been a result which, in turn, would have given reason for further action (now § 630 h, section 5, BGB).

The steadily rising number of reproaches heaped upon physicians for once reflects that patients are taking a more critical stand, which is basically not bad. The relative small number of physician condemnations in lawsuits for legal award on the other hand also speaks out for the eminent quality of medical services. It remains in the open though – or leaving something to argue about – whether the generation of the Patient Rights Act had truly been called for.

Explanation:
BGB = Bürgerliches Gesetzbuch: German Civil
*   Code*

Hospital Law in Germany and Europe

16

Christian Rybak and A. Moroder

Abstract

The legal framework for hospitals defines the functioning of hospitals' services as well as their financing and the financing of medical services carried out in the inpatient sector. The legal differentiation of this system succeeded the situation that hospitals have had problems to function in an economically successive way. The hospital financing is characterised by the DRG (diagnosis-related groups) system which means, in contrast to the outpatient sector, that medical services and all other hospital services are reimbursed in one-lump compensation.

The legal relationships between the hospital, patients and insurances are defined by the respective insurance membership of the patient. Social health insurances refund the costs for medical services directly to the hospital, whereas in the privately insured sector, the patient is cost debtor of the hospital and needs to get compensation by his insurance.

On the European scale, there do not exist specific provisions for hospitals because the legislative competence rests with the member states. However, there are some directives applicable to hospitals that concern specific security interests in the healthcare sector.

16.1 Introduction

Although the European community works more and more together in many economic and legal aspects, surprisingly there is no common medical law for the European Union.

Still all member states regulate medical issues by country specific law.

C. Rybak, LLD (✉) • A. Moroder
Wirtschaftsjurist (Univ. Bayreuth),
Widenmayerstraße 29,
Munich D-80538
Germany
e-mail: c.rybak@eep-law.de

© Springer-Verlag Berlin Heidelberg 2016
W. Merkle (ed.), *Risk Management in Medicine*, DOI 10.1007/978-3-662-47407-5_16

16.2 Overview

16.2.1 Legal Responsibilities from the Past Until Today

Understanding hospital law needs an insight into the developments of the past centuries. Today's sophisticated legal framework is a result of the professionalisation of the hospital structure and the general medical progress in Central Europe.

The history of hospitals starts with only patient care without a therapeutic setting. Well-known intellectuals and doctors entered hospitals and left their doctors' cabinets. With the foundation of the first university hospitals in the year 1710, the development of multidisciplinary centres started, in which medical diagnostics and therapies were carried out since then.

The request of hospital services is characterised by the medical progress, the introduction of the social health insurance system and the effects of the industrialisation and urbanisation of the beginning of the nineteenth century. Complex legal relations between social health insurances and hospitals developed. The basis has always been the principal of benefit (Sachleistungsprinzip) according to which the medical treatment was provided by the hospital to the patients without that the patient needs to fight for reimbursement.

Contracts between social health insurances and hospitals stood for the content of reimbursable medical treatment. State intervention and regulatory approaches started only in 1933 by the amendment of § 371 section 2 of the Reich Insurance Code (Reichsversicherungsordnung). The requirements for hospitals increased subsequently, and quality, hygiene and the service spectrum of medical care became more and more sophisticated.

A milestone for the German post-war period was the differentiation between municipal, independent and private hospital groups. At the same time, financial confrontations occurred. Hospital infrastructure was seen as public responsibility to be financed by taxpayers. However, modernisation and reconstruction measures were insufficient, and hospitals were seen as "Cinderella of the economic miracle".

Another milestone was the amendment of the German constitution of 12 May 1969 when article 74 no. 19a of the Constitution (Grundgesetz) was introduced. According to the latter, the competing legislation encompassed the economic security of hospitals and the regulation of the hospital payments. Hence, the Länder are in charge for the regulation of hospital infrastructure, and only the economic safety of hospitals was to be carried out by the Federal Government.

The Federal Government has regulated the financing of hospitals by the hospital finance act (Krankenhausfinanzierungsgesetz, KHG) of 19 June 1972. Furthermore, the reimbursement of hospital services was regulated by the responsibility for the social insurance system by the Federal Government. If hospitals are organised by church authorities, the organisation of those hospitals is regulated further by the freedom of religion, article 4 and 140 Grundgesetz.

Summing up, Germany knows a dual-finance system of hospitals that separates the hospital organisation by the Länder and the economic safety of hospitals by the Federal Government.

16.3 Definition of the Term "Hospital"

The hospital finance act (KHG) knows hospitals as institution, in which "medical and care services, diseases, damages are determined, cured or alleviated, obstetric care and in which patients are to be hosted and fed".

The relevant criterion to differentiate inpatient and outpatient care is the possibility of hosting and feeding and not the actual day and night care or hospitalisation. The definition also encompasses spa hospitals, preventive and rehabilitation institutions.

If companies want to run a private hospital, they need a specific concession of the competent authority according to § 30 of the trade regulation (Gewerbeordnung). They then can treat privately as well as publically insured patients according to the medical need. The definition of hospital care in private hospitals does not differ from the one mentioned above.

In recent times, mixed systems between in- and outpatient care have developed, and especially specialised care in hospitals according to § 116b of the Social Code Book V has broken the border between in- and outpatient care definitions.

16.4 Hospital Operators

Basically, German law knows three possible hospital operator types: public, independent and private ones. Public hospital owners are public bodies and establishments as well as foundations as, for example, the Federal Government, who, for example, runs military hospitals. Further, the Länder operate the university hospitals and municipal bodies operate public hospitals.

Secondly, private hospitals are operated by private hospital companies according to § 30 Gewerbeordnung. In Germany, one can observe increasing numbers of hospital companies as Rhön, Asklepios, Helios and Sana. Private hospitals are not supported financially according to the hospital financial act but operate on a market-oriented basis.

Third, independent hospitals are operated by the church or humanitarian or social associations as of, for example, the Red Cross. They are supported by the state but this does not mean the donation of money but only tax reductions.

16.5 Service Obligations of the Hospital

The spectrum of obligations for hospital doctors is regulated in both the German national hospital rate ordinance (Bundespflegesatzverordnung) and the German hospital fees act (Krankenhausentgeltgesetz). Also, § 39, 107 section 1 and 109 section 4 sentence 2 of the Social Code Book V regulate the spectrum of reimbursable hospital services. In order to obtain financial support, the hospital must be listed in the hospital plan which is determined by an official decision.

§ 8 section 1 sentence 4 KHEntG states literally that:

The public service of the hospital is deduced:

1. for the plan hospitals by the determinations of the hospital plan in connection with the official decisions for the implementation according to (…) the Hospital financing act as well as the accompanying agreement according to § 109 section 1 sentence 4 of the Social Code Book V.
2. For a university hospital by the recognition according to pathways regulated under Länder law, the hospital plan …
3. For other hospitals by the supply contract according to § 108 no. 3 of the Social Code Book V.

Other regulations are additionally determining what services are to be provided and to be reimbursed by the SHIs. § 39 of the Social Code Book V determines, for example, that insured patients may make use of hospital services and that they have to pay for any medically necessary hospital treatment that cannot be procured by outpatient doctors.

The public service obligation ("Versorgungsauftrag") of the hospital is defined by the assessment decision or the supply contract according to § 109 section 1 SGB V. The hospital plan, however, does not give the patient subjective public rates or duties. Only the location, the number of beds and the organisation of the hospital can be concluded from the hospital plan decision. The question on whether hospital services are to be paid for depends on whether hospital treatment is necessary. In the case of necessary inpatient treatment, the patient can demand the whole spectrum of medical services.

Thus, the hospital support depends on whether the hospital is listed in the hospital plan; in contrast to that, the reimbursement of medical services and the individual treatment need depends on the individual medical necessity.

If patients are not treated as they should and hospitals, for example, refuse to treat patients despite of the medical need, the Länder have the competence to supervise.

16.6   Hospital Financing

16.6.1 Dual Financing

The legal basis of the hospital financing is the hospital financing act (Krankenhausfinanzierungsgesetz, KHG). The purpose of the hospital financing is the economic security of hospitals and the supply of appropriate care.

The hospital financing act distinguishes between the support of hospital planning by the Federal Government, § 6 KHG, as well as the support of investment costs according to § 8 and 9 KHG. Further individual or global support is carried out by the Länder according to § 7 KHG. Furthermore, the economic safety of hospitals is to be carried out by nursing fees agreed by hospitals and social health insurances as well as the Länder (§ 17, 18, 18a KHG).

This system of dual financing of hospitals distinguishes between investment costs and operation costs of hospitals: The investment costs of hospitals are taken over by the Länder, whereas the operation costs are covered by the nursing fees and thus by the Federal Government.

It is sometimes unclear in the individual case whether costs are to be classified as investment or operation costs; there is a so-called Abgrenzungsverordnung to define and distinguish respective costs.

16.6.2 Hospital Financed Services in Detail

German hospital law knows the distinction between basic hospital services and optional services.

Basic hospital services are all medically necessary services in the individual treatment case, § 2 section 2 sentence 1 KHEntgG. These services are covered generally by fixed sum treatment amounts and additional fees. The latter equal the fee catalogue of § 7 section 1 KHEntgG that is applicable all over Germany.

Optional fees have to be paid for treatments that exceed medically needed services. It is obligatory to have an additional elective service agreement for those hospital matters in order to cover optional services. For example, optional services are the treatment by chief physicians or the accommodation in single or double bedrooms.

The hospital financing system is applicable for all hospitals that are included into the diagnosis-related group (DRG) system. Since 2004, the hospital financing by DRG is not optional anymore but obligatory. According to § 17b KHG, all medical treatments and services are to be coded by DRG numbers.

In general, hospitals are financed by yearly budgets agreed upon with the social health insurances. The institute for hospital reimbursement (INeK) calculates the reimbursement rates according to the case severity and the costs weights testified in the costs of the diagnosis-related groups. The mean effort of hospital services are displayed by the DRGs. The flat rates per case are establishing connection between the indication and diagnosis, the treatment and the time spent in the hospital.

16.7   Overview on the Law of Hospital Planning

Hospital planning is to be understood as requirements forecast for the hospitals and defines the requirements for performance capacities. The Länder are in charge for hospital planning, and they develop hospital plans according to § 6 KHG. Additionally, the Länder apply their own hospital laws which define the planning requirements for the respective Bundesland: this means the general (economic) goals as well as concrete regulations for the supply structures. Specifically, the Länder define the legal basis for the hospital planning, the content of the hospital plans and the realisation of the plan decisions and the respective procedure. These Länder regulations encompass the location of the hospital, the number of beds, the specialisations and the service level in different extent; for example, some Länder hospital laws only define the framework for hospital planning, whereas some regulate the hospital structures in detail.

16.7.1 Legal Character and Effect of the Hospital Plan

For hospitals, it is crucial to be part of the hospital plan because only hospitals listed are supported financially. Additionally, the commission of treating social health-insured patients depends on it. However, the amount of the compensation is regulated by the German ordinance on hospitalisation cost rate (Bundespflegesatzverordnung) and the annual agreements between hospitals and social health insurances as well as the Hospital Reimbursement Act (Krankenhausentgeltgesetz).

Legally, the hospital plan is an internal administrative matter without direct legal outward effect; especially, there is no possibility to object it by contradiction or legal action, not even for the payers.

In contrast to that, the individual decision for the respective hospital defines the requirements of the hospital planning. The single hospital has no legal right to be part of the hospital plan but only a right of justified decision on the uptake (ermessensfehlerfreie Entscheidung). Criteria are the capacity, the efficiency and the appropriateness of the hospital. Only in case that there is no alternative to the respective hospital, it must be uptaken into the hospital plan.

16.7.2 Content of the Hospital Planning

The goal of the hospital planning is adequate supplies of hospital services. The minimum content of the hospital planning is:

- Hospital goals
- Analysis of requirements
- Hospital analysis
- Definition of the service supply decision

In the end, the patients' needs of hospital supply are to be regulated in the hospital planning.

16.7.3 Identification of Needs

The service supply need of patients is to be calculated according to the Phil-Burton formulation. This formulation defines out of the assumed population, the hospital centralisation, the actual time spent in hospital and the use of beds per year what the need for hospital beds will be in the respective upcoming year. The calculation starts from the last year's figures:

$$\text{Planned beds} = \frac{\text{inhabitants} \times \text{hospital centralisation} \times \text{time spent in the hospital} \times 100}{1000 \times \text{use of beds} \times 365}$$

The hospital centralisation is counted as follows:

$$\text{Hospital centralisation} = \frac{\text{number of cases} \times 1000}{\text{Inhabitants}}$$

In fact, the identification of needs is subject to full judicial review.

16.8 Legal Aspects in Europe

Hospital law is not centralised within the EU, and the organisation of hospital supply is to be regulated by the member states according to art. 168 section 7 of the Treaty on the Functioning of the European Union (TFEU). The latter states that:

Union action shall respect the responsibilities of the Member States for the definition of their health policy and for the organisation and delivery of health services and medical care. The 26.10.2012 EN Official Journal of the European Union C 326/123 responsibilities of the Member States shall include the management of health services and medical care and the allocation of the resources assigned to them.

Thus, there do not exist hospital law regulations on a European level. However, there are some directives applicable for hospitals that concern specific security interests.

16.8.1 Directive EC 1235/2010: Pharmacovigilance

According to the directive EC 1235/2010, the pharmacovigilance system is equalised in Europe and the system for adverse reactions and the reporting of them is regulated consistently.

The European Medicines Agency analyses adverse reaction reports and creates a database (EudraVigilance). It is intended to make this database available to the public within the next years.

Consistently, the German Rules of Professional Practice for doctors regulate the obligation to report adverse reactions.

16.8.2 Directive EC 2000/34: EU Working Time Directive

According to the EU working time directive, hospitals need to respect minimum uninterrupted rest, minimum yearly holidays as well as weekly maximum working times and regulations for night and shift work.

However, there has been introduced a specific exception clause for hospitals aiming to guarantee continuity of patient care. According to the latter, any deviation of the working times needs to be adjusted by compensatory rest.

However, it was difficult to implement such a regulation, especially regarding the legal classification of stand-by services.

With decision of 03 October 2000, the ECJ decided that stand-by services are working times in case that doctors are spending the time in the hospital and not at home.

A revision of the EU Working Time Directive is in discussion but not in force yet.

16.8.3 Directive EC 2005/62: GCP for Blood and Blood Components

According to the directive EC 2005/62, the extraction and testing of human blood and blood components is regulated consistently for all member states. Good clinical practice for blood and blood components is thus harmonised. And the requirements for blood establishments are regulated on an EU level.

16.8.4 Directive EC 2010/32: Pinprick Directive

Pinpricks by needles or other sharp or pointed medical devices in the hospital sector are a severe infectious risk because of open wounds and blood contact. The pinprick directive regulates, for example, recapping, documentation of pinpricks as well as diminishing of the amount of sharp or pointed medical devices.

16.8.5 Directive EC 2013/55: Qualification Directive

Job qualifications are regulated in the qualification directive. Regarding the medical education, the directive regulates the requirements for basic medical training, the medical specialisation requirements as well as the education of nurses, midwives and pharmacists.

Hence, the recognition of job qualifications from abroad depends on whether the directives' requirements are met.

16.8.6 Directive 2013/59 Euratom: Protection from Radiological Contamination

Just recently, a new directive for radiological examinations has been approved that is intended to reduce the average exposure of radiation as well as the amelioration of the quality of radiological therapies.

Member states have to guarantee for:

- Training of people concerned with radiatic exposure.
- Procedures with the exposition of non-medical imaging have to be justified exceptionally.

- Regarding a medical exposition of nuclear material, the risk benefit assessment needs to be carried out every time.
- Reduction of radiatic exposure.
- Medical-physical experts are to be consulted if needed.
- Inventories need to be prepared for examining authorities.

Of course, there are further aspects of European law that influences the healthcare sector as of course the Pharmaceuticals Directive EC 2001/83. For hospitals, the above-mentioned aspects are of major interest despite of the lack of a European legal frame-work for hospitals: they do intervene the inpatient sector to a relevant extend although not directly treating the organization of hospitals.

Roger Roman Dmochowski

Abstract

Medical risk management in the United States remains a complicated process which involves not only an understanding of institutional experience but also regional as well as national expectations for outcomes and quality of care. Risk management requires integrated processes involving multiple aspects of institutional efforts including legal (general counsel) quality safety efforts, departmental and institutional leadership, as well as a formalized risk management group. Processes for identifying and analyzing present risk as well as potential future risk should be in place and formalized. These processes should be reproducible and be able to provide repetitive analyses that can be catalogued for purposes of tracking institutional experience and identifying environments within an institution that may be at risk for repetitive errors and/or risk-related activities

Risk management, as this concept pertains to medical care, is defined by a variety of activities that in aggregate will identify, mitigate, and reduce patient and/or health caregiver risk during the process of healthcare delivery. Other aspects of medical risk management involve mitigation of issues related to property and equipment misuse or damage and other contributors to financial threats to the individual institution. Risk management is defined by Mosby's Medical Dictionary as a "function of administration of a hospital or other health care facility directed toward identification, evaluation, and correct of potential risks that could lead to injury to patients, staff members, visitors or result in property damage of loss." Given the above considerations, there are multiple domains within risk management that identify, measure, mitigate, and resolve issues and/or circumstances that conspire to disrupt the above.

Within the surgical environment, risk management includes: activities not only related to surgery but also anesthesia, pre- and postoperative care, critical care, nursing, employment of appropriate and indicated technology, and factors related to hospital environment including

R.R. Dmochowski, MD, MMHC, FACS
Department of Urologic Surgery,
Vanderbilt University Hospital,
A1302 Medical Center North,
Nashville, TN 37232, USA
e-mail: roger.dmochowski@vanderbilt.edu;
ROGDEMO@AOL.COM

© Springer-Verlag Berlin Heidelberg 2016
W. Merkle (ed.), *Risk Management in Medicine*, DOI 10.1007/978-3-662-47407-5_17

infection control, overall safety, and the protection of employee rights.

In order for risk management to be appropriately performed, an infrastructure to support the aforementioned goals is critical. The "front lines" of risk management are the managers who are responsible for proactively identifying potential risks, establishing plans to mitigate risks, and implementing and monitoring those plans, algorithms, and protocols in an effort to minimize risk exposure.

Risk management cannot exist as an isolated function but must interact with general counsel (legal representing the institution) for purposes of litigation preparation and appropriate data acquisition. Specific support infrastructure should exist for purposes of identifying adverse events, cataloguing those events, and insuring evaluation of those events for purposes of process improvement. This activity requires interaction with an established and mature hospital quality and safety organization that should represent nursing and physician dyadic leadership.

Another aspect of risk management that is critical is preparation for mass casualty and other untoward events. Most institutions have emergency preparedness programs, and emergency preparedness should be fully integrated into risk management strategies and planning.

Certain types of hospitals will also engage in research activities that engender inherent risks and require not only surveillance but interaction of risk management with institutional review boards and institutional research entities for prevention and mitigation of events as they arise. A comprehensive risk management program will also interact with human resources (employee relations) to protect the physical and psychological welfare of individuals and detect concerns related to a hostile work environment or other workplace-based threats.

A critical aspect of risk management is the incorporation of open and transparent data acquisition, collection, monitoring, and reporting. Various institutions manage data acquisition differently. At Vanderbilt University Medical Center, the occurrences and concerns related to events are catalogued by an electronic reporting system. Any hospital employee or medical care provider (physician, nurse, assistant, technician, or student) may access the electronic reporting system in any area of the hospital. Event reports may be entered anonymously or with personal identification. The reports are categorized by the type of person entering the data, the time and date of the event, location, type of event (such as medication error, laboratory concern, behavioral event), others who may have witnessed or experienced the event, patient involved (if apropos including record identifying numbers), and finally a brief summary of the occurrence – if pertinent.

Once the report is entered, it is reviewed centrally by trained coding specialists within risk management who assess the accuracy and integrity of the report, reclassifying it as necessary. Depending upon the type of the report and the gravity of the risk associated, there is further review by risk management and involvement of centralized quality managers (who include representatives of both the medical and nursing leadership staff). The reports form the basis of a review strategy that is quite comprehensive.

For cases viewed as immediate and/or sentinel in nature, an event analysis (root cause analysis) is undertaken within a seven-day time frame to evaluate the specific event. Sentinel events include unexpected death, loss of life or limb, wrong site surgery, "never" events, death of child or mother in childbirth, and inhospital suicide. Less significant events that are deemed nonetheless significant after review by a combined committee including risk management and quality leadership will undergo adverse event analysis within 1 month of the occurrence for purposes of addressing systems and other issues that may have contributed to the event.

Event analysis groups include trained risk managers, trained quality consultants, the members of the team who were involved with specific incident, as well as direct supervisors. Additionally, other support personnel are present as needed including human resources and general counsel. The event analysis follows a prespecified method of assessment that includes initial discussion of the actual event and then each individual's remembrance of the occurrences that led to the event. Where appropriate, systems engineers will assess for human factors that may have contributed to the event for purposes of managing system flaws and/or system-based risks. Event analyses are focused on system-based concerns; however, individual contribution to the event is also assessed, and when medical care provider concerns are identified, peer review may be initiated. Similarly, if nonprovider (such as technician) contribution to an event is identified, human resource (employee ombudsman) input may also be included. Once the event analysis is completed, the analytic report is reviewed by senior leadership and then agreed-upon strategies and/or tactics for managing that risk and any future risk are agreed upon, and planning and management for strategic change are enacted.

One other category of event is immediately managed in conjunction with human resources and institutional leadership. This category of event is one in which a boundary violation occurs such as sexual or racial harassment, physical or mental abuse, or hostile or threatening behavior. Physical violence and/or other implied or real threats also fall into this mandated or egregious category. Immediate intervention is undertaken with the individuals, both who received the aggression and also the individual who undertook the aggression. There is a strict algorithm for intervention for the egregious/mandated acts that exists and has been agreed upon by institutional leadership for purposes of redress of the circumstances that led to the event.

This robust process allows rapid and systematized approaches to adverse or untoward events in a manner that can contribute to rapid cycle improvement and mitigation of any subsequent risks. Clearly, timeliness of response to adverse event is critical, especially given the potential for subsequent similar events. Institutional leadership must be in consonance with the management methods established for adverse event recognition, evaluation, and response. Without leadership agreement and support, these programs will not succeed (Fig. 17.1).

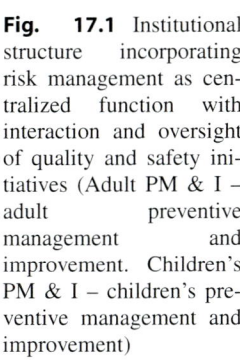

Fig. 17.1 Institutional structure incorporating risk management as centralized function with interaction and oversight of quality and safety initiatives (Adult PM & I – adult preventive management and improvement. Children's PM & I – children's preventive management and improvement)

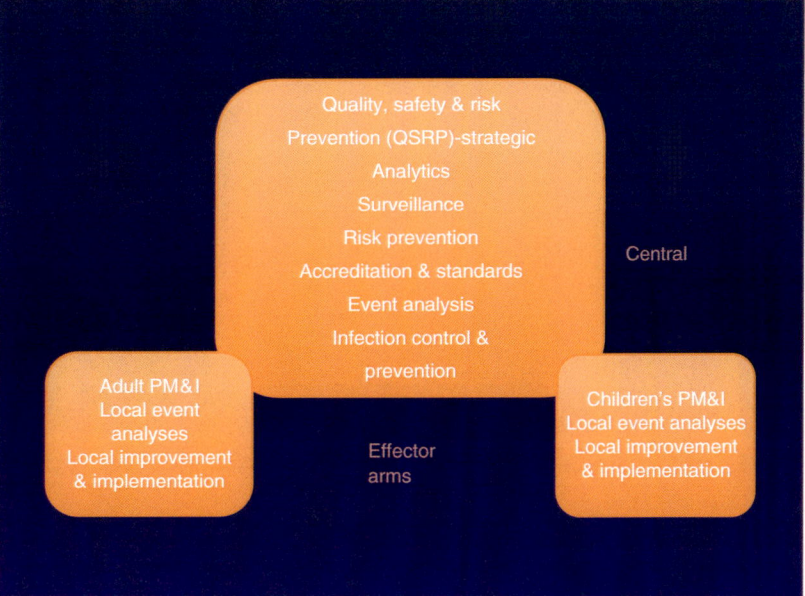

Insurance Problems

18

R.A. Patrick Weidinger

Abstract

Within the existing systems of the liability insurance, financial constructs will not be able to limit the number of claims and the claims amount.

A change in the system towards a state-controlled patient insurance would not correspond to the interests of victims who suffered iatrogenic damages to receive comprehensive compensation at current levels.

This is why the solution can only be a comprehensive and constant risk management process.

18.1 The Problems Encountered and Tasks to Be Resolved by Liability Insurers in Germany

The task of the liability insurance entails the investigation of the question of liability insurance, the rejection of unjustified claims and the financing of valid damage claim liabilities.

The insurance companies in Germany organised in the form of public limited companies must ensure that indemnity payments do not permanently exceed the premiums collected by the insurance company as this would lead to such companies becoming insolvent. If the insurance company provides insurance for a hospital or individual physicians, a forecast of the course of the insured financial year, e.g. the year 2015, has to be calculated. Here, contrary to the insurance of vehicles, the insurer will encounter a number of unforeseeable events. For an insurance in accordance with "occurrence" (a common principle in Germany), the insurer has to ascribe any and all damages to the year 2015 that have taken place in 2015, although such damages might only be reported to the insurer at a later date, but as a rule the insurer will only know in the year 2025 how successful or unsuccessful that year has been (one only needs to think about artificial hip replacements implanted incorrectly and breaking in the year 2022). The insurance in accordance with "claims made" carries an analogue risk for damages incurred by the end of the year 2014, unless the insurer has defined a retroactive date (please see chapter 18 III 2). In Germany we need to add to this long-tail topic a further point[1]: the costs for large claims like hypoxic

R.A.P. Weidinger
Abteilungsldirektor,
Deutsche Ärzteversicherung Aktiengesellschaft,
Martinstr. 9A, Wiesbaden 65189, Germany
e-mail: patrick.weidinger@aerzteversicherung.de

[1] Hellberg/Lonsing deliver new information for the calculation and reserving processes in hospitals, VersWi

brain damage after a delayed sectio caesarea, incorrect intubation, anaphylactic shock etc. are increasing to such an extent that the insurance premiums have reached dimensions in the field of gynaecology with obstetrics that the clients of the insurer can no longer afford these premiums. Due to the complexity of the topic, many insurers have left the field of insurance for physicians and hospitals.

18.2   Situation Outside of Germany

The problems described here are also known to liability insurers outside of Germany.[2] At this point, we would like to remind you of the discussions held in other European countries and the insurance crisis that took place in the United States of America.[3] A difference to such structures is to be found in countries where all of the social security matters are covered by the State, as, for example in New Zealand where a national accident insurance and in Scandinavia where a patients' insurance prevails.[4]

18.3   Why Is It That the Insurances Cannot Offer Financial Solutions

1. Deductibles of the insurance client to serve a limitation of the claims expenditure do not make much sense. These would only make sense in the case of large claims if the amount would run up to a noticeable amount of EUR 500,000.00 and more.[5] However, many insured parties cannot afford such figures.

2. In the field of General Liability Insurance and in accordance with German Law, the decisive moment for the insurer and the temporal responsibility of the insurer is the point in time of the occurrence of the damage (occurrence). The Anglo-American system however takes into account the point in time of the claim (claims made).[6] Claims-made has the advantage for the insurer that he does not have to calculate long-tail risks as he is not responsible for damages incurred after the insurance term but rather the subsequent insurer. However, this advantage will be lost again by a subsequent change to the loss event system as the claims-made insurer has to offer secondary liability insurance. This is possibly also the reason why the claims-made package has not yet been established in Germany.[7]

3. This means that the insurance premium has to be calculated in such a way that the amount of coverage of the company has a positive result. The calculation basis is the claims history from which a forecast will result on the basis of certain mathematical procedures like chain ladder, taking also into consideration any belated claims (IBNR – incurred but not reported). The premiums for a hospital can be calculated in accordance with different models, for example, in the form of premiums according to beds, sales or cases. Due to a declining number of beds available in clinics and the reduced time of stay in hospitals, the former defining number of beds is no longer an appropriate measure. Nowadays priority is given to calculations based on sales. Yet all of these calculation models are to be looked at as crutches conveying apparent safety and plausibility to the client. In the end, it does not matter which model has been chosen, the goal must always be profitability. The calculation

---

13/2012, 62 ff.

[2] Please see L'ARGUS DE L'ASSURANCE vom 15.04.05, Seite 38 ff: Assurances RC Médicale: Un mal francais?

[3] Details: (1) Krahe, Die Haftungssystematik bei ärztlicher Arbeitsteilung und Zusammenarbeit in den Vereinigten Staaten von Amerika und in Deutschland, ISBN 3-89820-756-0, (2) Flatten, Die Arzthaftpflichtversicherung in den Vereinigten Staaten von Amerika, ISBN 3-631-30699-7.

[4] Weidinger in Ehlers/Broglie, Arzthaftungsrecht, Kapitel 4 (5 Auflage 2013).

[5] Weidinger, Versicherungswirtschaft 2005, 1332.

[6] Weidinger in Wenzel, Fachanwalt Medizinrecht, Kapitel 5, Rdnr. 194 ff. m.w.N.

[7] Weidinger in Wenzel, Der Arzthaftungsprozess Kapitel 2 B II 1 b m.w.N.

risks result from statistically speaking incidental claims, from the mathematically speaking low number of actual claims and the constantly changing environment. These factors do not only affect the development in medicine and law but also the equipment and changes in the field of human resources in hospitals.

18.4   Risk Management and Claims Prevention Through the Insurance Business

It has been the experience of the author[8] that in manageable closed systems such as in individual hospitals, declining claims must be generated soon. The implementation of quality management mainly occurs in accordance with the principle PDCA (plan, do, check, act).

Essential elements of such a risk management are among others the financial review and

---

[8] The author can look back on 25 years of experience gathered in managerial functions in the German insurance business covering a claims portfolio of 3000–7000 iatrogenic claims per year.

analysis of all claims made during the last 15 years, the validation of all processes and of the quality management and the implementation of standards (e.g., admission of the patient, treatment, patient information, documentation, guidelines, the dual control system, learning from mistakes, CIRS).

• Introduction of controlling
• Half-yearly meetings with hospital physicians about future potential
• The development of constantly updated codes of practice (including what to do in the case of claims)

18.5   Summary

Within the existing systems of the liability insurance, financial constructs will not be able to limit the number of claims and the claims amount.

A change in the system towards a state-controlled patient insurance would not correspond to the interests of victims who suffered iatrogenic damages to receive comprehensive compensation at current levels.

This is why the solution can only be a comprehensive and constant risk management process.

Implementation of Risk Management in Hospitals

19

Patrik Herrscher and Andreas Goepfert

Abstract

This book shows you that both, legal and other factors, can be necessary to implement a risk management system in clinic. The company management must intensively consider the issue and develop a risk strategy for the clinic. First a project plan and a pilot area are needed, in which the clinic would start to integrate risk management. After all basics have been created and a risk manager is introduced, the risk management process is carried out in a first risk inventory, which includes documentation of risks and measures. The risk management cycle is repeated continuously, to ensure monitoring of risks and adaptation of activities. If the system is established, it applies this to evaluate and implement necessary improvement measures. A risk management manual documents rules and responsibilities within the system. Finally, risk management should be monitored at regular intervals by an independent auditor.

19.1 Main Reason for Implanting a Risk Management System in Hospitals

In the past few years, clinical risk management is getting more and more important for hospitals. The reasons for this are increased patient confidence and higher willingness to fight by law when errors of a medical treatment might be possible. Other reasons are that risk management can reduce costs and prevent from losing the image, when errors in treatment are getting published. Apart from this, there are legal requirements that make the introduction of risk management necessary. As an example, the German law on control and transparency in business (KonTraG) says in § 91 AktG (stock law): "The board shall take appropriate measures,

P. Herrscher (✉)
Leiter Dienstleistungszentrum Qualitäts-
und Risikomanagement, ANregiomed,
Escherichstr. 1, Ansbach 91522, Germany
e-mail: p.herrscher@vkla.de

A. Goepfert, MD
ANregiomed,
Escherichstr. 1, Ansbach 91522, Germany
e-mail: a.goepfert@vkla.de

© Springer-Verlag Berlin Heidelberg 2016
W. Merkle (ed.), *Risk Management in Medicine*, DOI 10.1007/978-3-662-47407-5_19

in particular to establish a monitoring system to ensure the continuation of the Company's dangerous developments early be recognized." Further this law regulates that risk management system should be checked regularly and must be a part of a check report. The report hast to give an answer on the question if the management has taken all actions to introduce an appropriate risk management system. In addition to the statutory requirements, a risk management system is also needed in standards such as the DIN EN 15224 or the ISO 9001 norm. Certification schemes – for example in Germany KTQ – often require a risk management system. In the growing patient information portals within the Internet, safety indicators are transparent and understandable to the public.

19.2   General

Important for the implementation of a risk management system is to realize that there are a variety of risks in hospitals, resulting from treatment and care of patients and to know that there are many of processes to support that.[1] Everywhere people are working, there is the possibility of errors (Chap. 1). This risk is applicable in all areas and should be kept as low as possible and detected as fast as possible, so that the negative effects remain small and can be intercepted by suitable measures. In the previous book chapters, the risk management tools have been intensively discussed, so that they shall not be dealt in this chapter. The aim of this book chapter is giving the reader a clear guide to handle for the implementation of a risk management system in a hospital.

19.3   Implementation of a Risk Management

19.3.1 Planning the Project and Project Kick Off

In the first step, the project must be planned. An important part of the planning is to calculate the

financial and human resources for the project. It must also be thought about external consultants in the project and whether they are needed or not. Another planning step is to define a pilot area for risk management, which can definitely make sense in larger hospitals. The intension on that is that problems in the start-up phase can be solved in a small starting area which has normally less barriers than starting in the whole company. As soon as the project planning is completed, it is very important to inform the managers about the project, the plan, the need for risk management and the associated costs. This can take place, for example, in the form of a kickoff event. Clear communication of the high priority of this project is important, and associated benefits must be pointed out.

19.3.2 Developing the Risk Strategy

As soon as the executives are informed about the project, it is important that the management strictly is engaged supporting the risk strategy. This can take place together with the employees or managers in workshops. In an increasingly competition between hospitals, it is important to realize opportunities while deciding where are the risks. Risk management is a management function, and head of hospital should pursue the desired goal with vigor and communicate this in the company clear and unambiguous. For this purpose, sufficient resources must be provided and the construction process of a risk-conscious corporate culture must be promoted.

19.3.3 Organizational Structure for Risk Management

First of all, the construction of risk management in the clinic must be defined. Figure 19.1 shows a possible configuration of the system.

Essential elements in the organization structure of the risk management system, as shown in Fig. 19.1, are the risk owners in the departments and the risk manager. Consequently, the next step in the implementation of risk management is to employ a risk manager for the clinic and then to appoint risk owners of the departments.

---

[1] Mentzel: Risikomanagement im Krankenhaus. In: Zapp, Winfried (Hg.): Risikomanagement in Stationären Gesundheitseinrichtungen. Heidelberg 2011, S. 202.

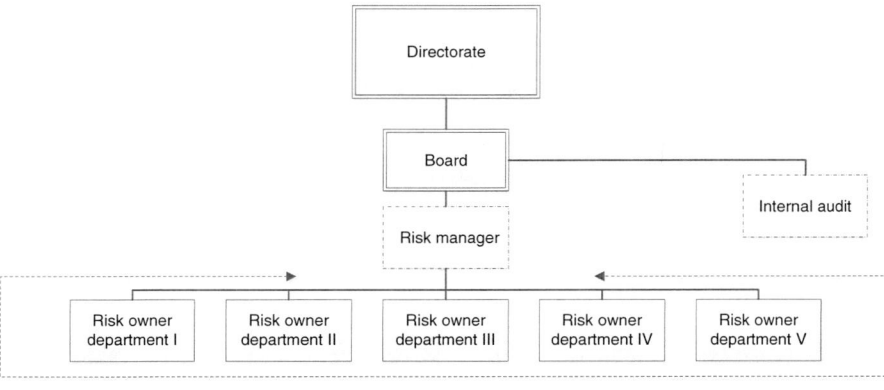

Fig. 19.1 Example of an organizational structure (Source: own presentation)

19.3.4 Implementation of Risk Manager

The risk manager is the central hub of the system and ensures that the system is living. Without a person who directs the system and, if necessary, takes corrective action and demanding an implementation with long-term existence is inconceivable. The risk manager is the central point of contact within the company for risks and provides communication between the board, the management, and the risk owners. His responsibilities include the following among others:

- Training of employees.
- Detecting/identifying and analyses of risks and errors.
- Evaluate and report risks.

Cases evaluation

- Advising management.
- Moderating working and project groups.
- Perform the risk inventory check.

Employees for this job, for example, can be acquired from quality management, since the quality management of a clinic in most cases already includes components of clinical risk management. The position of risk manager should be connected as a staff position at the company's management to perform its tasks effectively. Because resources are often scarce in the clinics, it should in principle be considered whether the

quality and risk management cannot be closely linked, and therefore the task of the risk manager may be perceived by the quality management of the clinic. Because of the specific knowledge of the risks and the dangers in the departments, the risk manager needs some persons called risk owners in the departments. The responsibility for the control and monitoring of the risks lies with the leaders in the fields of nursing, medicine, and administration. Often clinics have difficulty in assigning the risks of a business executive. In such case, it is necessary that an assignment held by the management is implemented. In no case, inconsistencies and jurisdictional disputes are resolved within the risk management system.[2]

19.3.5 IT Support

Another important decision is the way how risks are documented and reported. Since there are a variety of risks from different areas in a hospital and all departments should involve, IT support for documentation, monitoring, and reporting is almost mandatory in order to keep the effort for all involved as low as possible. It is important to respect it, that the software is user-friendly and intuitive to us. Preference should be given to solutions that can be found Web based to enable

---

[2] Jakob/Richter: Integriertes Risikomanagement – Mehr als nur eine Pflichtübung. In: Zapp, Winfried (Hg.): Risikomanagement in Stationären Gesundheitseinrichtungen. Heidelberg 2011, S. 301.

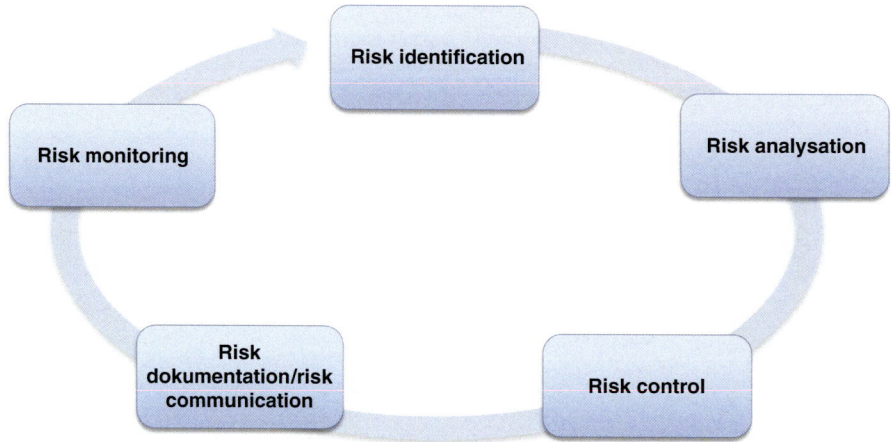

Fig. 19.2 Risk management process (Source: own presentation)

access from different locations, platforms, and users. A client software version focuses the identification of risks and the maintenance of the software exclusively on a single computer or on a limited number of clients, which also need to be maintained by the IT department. Other issues that should be brought in connection with the acquisition are costs and benefits, administrative expenses, the rights and role of management, possible interfaces to the KIS, and the range of analysis options.[3]

19.3.6 Tasks and Training of Risk Owners

Each risk owner is responsible for monitoring and early detection of risks in his own area. He identifies and analyzes risks and reports them an hoc to the risk manager.[4] For this reason, it is necessary to teach the risk owner in basics of the risk management system. This training should be as practical as possible introducing the risk owners in handling risk management tools in their own departments.

19.3.7 Risk Management Process

The actual risk management process is divided into five phases and is understood as a cycle. Figure 19.2 shows the circuit graphically.

The following text should serve giving the reader an approach to their hand, as the risk management process can be practically implemented in the clinic. All steps presuppose that all participants in the risk management process and the procedure in the company are known.

19.3.7.1 First Step Risk Identification

A long-term goal must be that the identification of risks is a part of the daily work of staff and that all employees see it as their entire duty to point out these risks and to report all(!) of them.

There are two types of risk identification: first experience-based methods (regressive methods). These are deriving risks from occurring cases of damage or injury. On the other analytical methods, they serve to identify risks already in the development phase[5] (Chap. 11). A mixture of both methods is also known as risk inventory analysis. In this case, an inventory of risks in each area is triggered by the risk manager in a certain temporal rhythm. First, this should take

---

[3] Jakob/Richter 2011.

[4] Gleißner: Grundlagen des Risikomanagements im Unternehmen. München 2011, 2., Auflage, S. 247.

[5] Conrad: Klinisches Risikomanagement. Münster 2006, 2. Auflage, S. 98.

place in the designated pilot area. In general a well prepared first inventory of an area takes approximately 3–4 h to complete. Here, the risk manager loads the risk officers from one or more areas and acquires a dialog risks. Often it is not easy to identify the potential risks in their area clearly – even not for risk managers. Because of that, it has proved to give example risk categories as a support to make risk adjustment available. The following risk categories can be used among others as possible starting points in clinics:

- Market (competitors, referrers)
- Legal framework (laws, environmental laws, hospital financing, labor laws)
- Infrastructure (IT, supply, waste disposal, communication, technology, logistics)
- Staff (cost increase, bottleneck, fluctuation, etc.)
- Finance (increasing costs, shortfalls, interest rate risks, investment, tax, liability)
- Buildings (construction projects, security, fire, contaminated sites, renovation)
- Communication (media, image, crises)
- Purchase (price increases, supplier relationships, procurement constraints, contracts, announcement)
- Medicine (treatment failure, medicine technologies, care, processes, rehabilitation)
- Environment (storms, landslides, epidemics)
- Company (hygiene, organizational structure, data protection, working security, organization)

Internal and external reports, CIRS reports, error collection lists, or direct tip by employees can clue more about potential risks. They must also be addressed in the risk inventory.

19.3.7.2 Risk Assessment

Once the risks have been identified, it is necessary to carry out an assessment of risks in order to get a more accurate idea about how serious this is and what effects to expect of it (Chap. Risikobewertung). The assessment of risks is the central focus of risk management, because only risks are identified and evaluated; it is possible to control them in the next step.[6] The risk assessment can be part of the risk inventory. In a dialog, the risk owner and the risk manager are talking about the expected level of damage and the possible occurrence probability in a specific time period. The product of possible monetary loss and probability of occurrence is referred to as loss expectancy. This is a measure that provides an average value over the expected damage from the risk.[7] The determination of the amount of loss is certainly not easily possible because the damage cannot be clearly calculated in monetary form. Such a risk may be, for example, a loss of image due to hygiene deficiencies. No one can predict how many patients, because of such an incident, avoid temporarily or even permanently to look for treatment in this hospital. In such a case, it makes sense – nevertheless to use estimates for any possible damage – to clearly identify the risk in the company and to make it visible. Simply and clearly, this process is shown by a visual representation of risks within a risk matrix (risk map) (Fig. 19.3).

The illustrated two-dimensional matrix includes a total of 25 individual fields in which the risks can be classified. The third dimension is recognizable by the expected loss, which are, as described above, the product of probability and extent of damage. Depending on the expected loss, the risk can be divided into different levels, which should be defended depending on the monetary value of damage during the risk strategy formation by the company management. In case classification on the monetary or percentage values is problematic, the literal gradations can be used as an aid to still achieve a classification and localization of the risk in the risk matrix. The risk matrix additionally serves to simplify the comparison between the risks and thus uncover particularly threatening risk.

---

[6] Ritschl: Herausforderungen des Risikomanagements im Krankenhaus. Hamburg 2012, S. 14.

[7] Katarzyna: Optimierung eines Risikomanagementsystems im Mittelstand. Norderstedt 2009, S. 52.

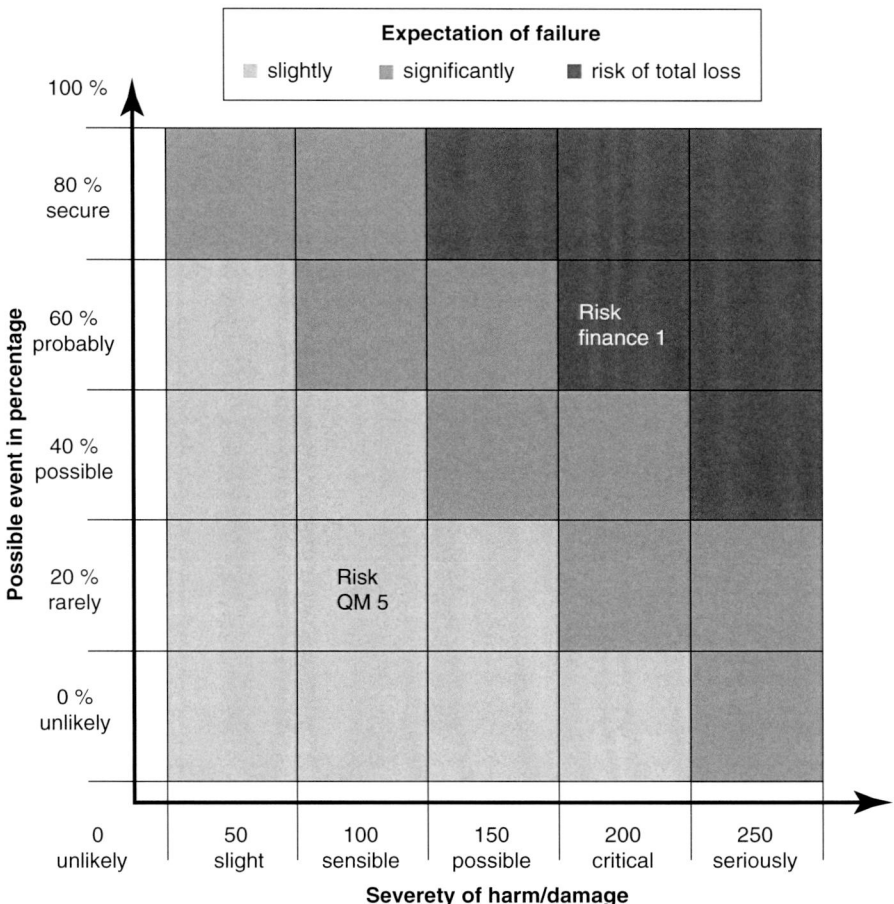

Fig. 19.3 Risk map (Source: own presentation)

19.3.7.3 Risk Control

Identified and evaluated risks must be controlled. A query which already initiated countermeasures may take place parallel to the risk inventory and can also be documented in the IT solution. To manage the risks, there are four strategies:

Risk avoidance: It tries to avoid the risk of special products that can be dangerous.

Risk reduction: Can be achieved, for example, by teaching employees, using clinical pathways, or coordinating processes and interfaces between departments.

Risk transfer: For example, to transfer the financial risk to an insurance company if possible

or source out some serious work to experts of an external company.

Risk prevention or carrying the risk itself: The risk is accepted and supported by the company.

All risks that exist after measures and in the worst case carried by the company are named as net risks.[8] In the controlling of risks, it is important to name specific individuals responsible for each risk, which direct the actions and the risk documentation

---

[8] Graebe-Adelssen: Risk Management – die Sicht von außen. In: Graf et al. (Hrsg.) Risk Management im Krankenhaus – Risiken begrenzen und Kosten steuern, 2003, S. 23.

of the given situation. As risks often affect not just one area, it is also useful to set up a kind of steering committee for risk management, which links the different areas on to the other.

19.3.7.4 Risk Documentation and Communication

Risk communication about the risks and its documentation are important steps leading all stakeholders to be aware of the risk issue. Optimally this creates a new risk consciousness that leads to a self-perpetuating process, thus new risks will be reported to the risk manager immediately.

The risk report is an essential part of risk management. This serves the risks to staff, risk owners, board, and other interested parties; thus, risks by priority order are shown as clear as possible. In the best case, the hospital has decided in advance to install software for risk management that generates a report by one button click and allows various report designs for the different stakeholders. If this is not the case, we must consider how to document the risks most clearly. An open access excel sheet might be an alternative. But this only works for small clinics. It is not possible to set individual read and write permissions, access ways, and copy limits, so that the table in most cases would have to be maintained by the risk manager as well.

19.3.7.5 Risk Monitoring

The previous step of the documentation and reporting is closely linked to the risk monitoring. In regular intervals, the status of the individual risk should be verified by the risk owners and analyzed for possible changes. This can take place in the form of a renewed risk inventory, prompting the risk managers at certain intervals, which may be, for example, quarterly or semiannually. Actually how far the measures take effect can often be assessed only afterwards. If improperly performed or no actions taken as an adverse impact on the company, the benefits of the risk

management system is often difficult to moor in numbers. A regular monitoring of all risks and associated actions will always lead to the fact that nothing is lost of what could be jeopardizing the continued existence under the specific circumstances of the clinic.

19.4 Risk Management Manual

As part of the risk management system, the risk manual covers many documents and records, which describe all important points and make it transparent for all employees . Furthermore, it is important that the individual actors in the system are clearly identified and the roles and responsibilities are described in the manual. The finished manual is not a rigid set of rules but should rather be a living documentation of the system that is continually revised and improved under the supervision of the risk manager.

19.5 Monitoring by an Independent Auditor

At regular intervals, the entire process of risk management must be illuminated by an independent test to detect possible system problems. An internal audit may serve as for independent inspection.

The main tasks include:

- Controlling the compliance of all regulations in risk manual
- Discovering possible gaps and uncovered vulnerabilities
- Assessing practicability of the system
- Identifying potential for improvement

An independent assessment can also be guaranteed by certification, for example, on the basis of an extern annual audit; see Chap. 21 for details.

19.6 Summary

Both legal and many other external and internal factors make it necessary to implement a hospital-wide risk management. For this purpose, the management must seriously address the issue and develops a risk strategy for the clinic. In the next step, a project planning must take place, which, according to hospital size, initially integrates a pilot area in the start of risk management. All the basics are in place and the risk management process is called a risk manager carried out in a first inventory risk with the risk owners of the departments and document the risks and measures. The risk management cycle is repeated continuously to ensure monitoring of risks and adaption measures. A risk management manual decremented duties and responsibilities within the system and provides the necessary transparency in the processes for all employees. If system is established, it should be checked at regular intervals by an independent auditor to identify improvement potentials and promote the system in terms of the continuous improvement process.

Economic Aspects of Risk Management: Introduction to RM and CIRS in Hospital as an Economic Task Based on a Practical Example

20

Rainer Riedel and Aliki Schmieder

Abstract

Although there is already a high level of medical patient care in Germany, it is of interest for patients, medical staff, hospital owners, and liability insurance to be aware of potential medical malpractice at an early stage using an integrated Critical Incident Reporting System (CIRS).

The authors follow the question how far the German hospitals have introduced a defined risk management system (RM) showing possible hospital needs to establish a risk management system. On the basis of these results, hospital managers in other countries can benchmark their own risk prevention systems with the German model.

On the basis of a model hospital, the practical implementation of RM and CIRS should be proved.

In the context of this risk management project, the focus was directed to the surgery wards – as a department with the highest potential for value creation – aimed to analyze the pathways along the perioperative process to test for inefficiencies and to illuminate the sub-processes from the perspective of possible emerging risks.

The error-prone problem areas were identified, and the sub-process steps were adjusted by risk management aspects.

The introduction of CIRS was carried out as an integral part of the project which follows a clearly defined project plan taking into account the recommendations on the German Alliance for Patient Safety.

With the introduction of the RM and this CIRS model, the hospital aims to establish a sustainable improvement of patient safety. From the author's point of view, this must be accompanied by a confidence building clinic culture, which should be developed continuously.

R. Riedel, MD, PhD (✉)
Institut für Medizin-Ökonomie,
Medizinische Versorgungsforschung – iMÖV,
Schaevenstr. 1a-b, Köln 50676, Germany
e-mail: riedelkoeln@gmx.de

A. Schmieder, MA
Masterstudiengang Medizinökonomie,
RFH Köln, Schaevenstr. 1a-b,
Köln 50676, Germany
e-mail: aliki.schmieder@netcologne.de

© Springer-Verlag Berlin Heidelberg 2016
W. Merkle (ed.), *Risk Management in Medicine*, DOI 10.1007/978-3-662-47407-5_20

20.1   Introduction

Patient safety is the primary focus of medical and nursing actions (primum nihil nocere); despite utmost care medical malpractice and secondary failures cannot always be avoided in the treatment of patients – although physicians and nursing staff are concerned about working as fault free as possible. If faults happen, it is in the nature of man and of the existing fault culture that they do not like to talk about their faults openly: The responsible persons tend to reduce the damaging event to a possible human failure and impose sanctions. This form of fault management uses these respective opportunities to learn from their mistakes in *a very specified way*!

Nevertheless, can we really learn from third parties? Today, the answer to this question is without any doubt "yes." For several decades already, international aviation people learn from narrow escapes as well as from actual mistakes that occur within the "system of learning" from each other.

As a result, there is a definite need to analyze the causes of patient-related incidents and secondary damages of patients, regardless of medical or nursing actions. A risk analysis behind the causes in the hospital routine arrives at the conclusion that the potential source of faults does not trace back to an individual employee but instead to the existing methodical procedures.

Now, in the period of the patients' rights law, it is in the interest of patients, medical staff, hospital owners, and liability insurance to identify sources of potential medical malpractice at an early stage by means of an internal clinic RM system with an integrated Critical Incident Reporting System (CIRS). Thus, an appropriate management process focusing on the patient care should be implemented (Riedel et al. 2013). *Please see relevant sections of the book* (Chaps. 1, 5, 6, and 9).

Irrespective to the discussion improving the safety of patients and employees by implementing an RM system, it should be mentioned that there is already a high level of medical patient care in Germany; however, this fact should not prevent the lowering of the existing fault rate in relation to the interest of individual patients and the medical staff.

On the basis of a benchmark hospital, the practical implementation of RM and CIRS will be represented. This benchmark hospital focuses on medical care, with a "central OP" with five OP rooms and 400 beds.

The hospital is KTQ certified, and within the framework of the audit, the auditor harshly criticized the unsufficiently documented fault management as an integral part of the RM system because of the missing CIRS. Consequently, the management of the hospital planned and realized an implementation of a CIRS.

First of all, the question is why a hospital needs to establish an RM system? This discussion is conducted regularly in hospitals. However, a few private companies have recognized the benefits of a working RM and are systematically building appropriate structures that support the *group clinics* to implement this RM process faster and finally successfully. It is clear that this concerted approach has a lot of advantages, e.g., by mutual use of peer review processes, and therefore the economic profit becomes evident for the implementation of RM (*see also* Chap. 19).

20.2   RM and Its Position in the Hospital

An RM is an essential element within every responsible company management (Krystek and Fiege 2013). In this way, there is no distinction between industrial enterprises and hospitals. Without a functioning RM, the existence of the company is jeopardized in case of the worst case scenario which could have been prevented by using RM system.

The RM subsumes the dealing with all the risks that might arise or occur, respectively, in a company such as a clinic. This also means the risks arising inside the "company" hospital itself, e.g., road safety obligation (grit the road in case of black ice, etc.), hazardous substance maintenance (radioactive substances, gases, infectious waste, etc.), or computer problems (data safety, etc.) (*see also* Chap. 1). In accordance with the

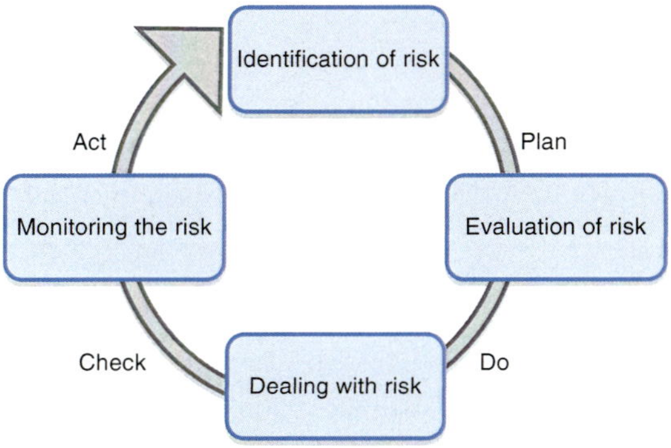

Fig. 20.1 RM process represented according to the PDCA cycle (Source: own figure)

RM process, potential risks and faults are systematically identified then in the second step are analyzed and prevented, and consequently, in the third step, actions are taken to deal with them. Finally, one has to evaluate these RM preventing measurements during the fourth step. The entire process is a subject to a continuous improvement cycle which basically corresponds to the PDCA cycle (*see* Chap. 6, Fig. 20.1).

It should be kept in mind that a proactive implementation of an effective RM system in a hospital requires a new transparency to deal with the possibilities of medical malpractice. A sanction must be avoided, and one should learn from the near misses of the past to avoid them in the future.

This also implies a new future-oriented hospital organizational culture which in the medium term will lead to new forms of team orientation, particularly for the doctors and nursing staff. Only if traditional service structures can be overcome can this be clearly implemented, for example, by means of well-founded communication. Such an approach also has its effects in the personnel planning process considering qualification and structural organization.

Basically, one has to be aware that an RM system may not only lead to the improvement of patient safety; such a system is also an important mechanism for the protection of the employees themselves in the hospital. At the end of the day, only a low-risk hospital is able to secure its economic survival in the long-term avoiding expensive patient liability cases.

Also keep in mind – concerning such medical faults which were committed by an employee of the hospital – that they might suffer significant psychological stress and/or strain from a given medical malpractice, that, e.g., for doctors sometimes, such cases end up of being revoked from further practice of their profession. In view of the tense labor market, especially with its shortage of nursing staff and doctors, a working RM system is an important factor for an attractive working environment in a hospital.

Attention should be paid especially to the following risks:

- Points of intersection (admission, discharge, shift change, change of ward)
- Nosocomial infection
- Polypharmacotherapy
- Tumbles
- Mistaken identity (patient/tests, diagnostic findings, identification)
- Diagnostic fault
- Surgical fault
- Emergency treatment for stationary admitted patients
- Correct operation of fielding medical technology

At present, the benchmark hospital can use the following sources for risk identification fields:

(a) *Internal sources:*
    - Analysis of medical report
    - Complaint management
    - Analysis of patient claims and/or beneficiaries
    - Field data (direct observation of clinical processes)
    - Mortality and morbidity conference
    - External and internal risk audits
    - Patient questioning
    - Analysis of data for accounting or external quality assurance
    - Analysis of own key figures (readmission rate, number of tumbles, statistics on infected wounds, revision rate)

(b) *External sources:*
- Liability insurance references
- Information about CIRS professional organizations (CIRS-AINS, PASOS, CIRS Medical)
- Benchmarking the QM structures *in comparison to other hospitals*
- Hospital quality reports

The legal regulations in recent years show that the need to establish an RM system is not a new challenge.

In fact, the need for RM has arisen from a series of legal provisions that came more into focus over the years (Krystek and Fiege 2013), such as:

- *IDW PS 340* (1998): Examination of the system for early risk detection according to § 317 section 4 of German Commercial Code
- Act for Control and Transparency in the Corporate Sector (*KonTraG*) (1998)
- Sarbanes-Oxley-Act (2002)
- Requirements of the German Corporate Governance Codex (*DCGK*) (2002)
- Accounting Law Modernization Act (*BilMoG*) (2009)
- Minimum Requirements for RM (*MaRisk*) (*BA*), International Financial Reporting Standards (*IFRS*) (2009)
- *ISO Norm 31000:* Standard for RM (2009)
- *Infektionsschutzgesetz:* Act on the protection against infections (2001, latest amendment 08/2013)
- *Patientenrechtegesetz:* Patients' Rights Law (2013)

In particular, the BGB (Civil Code) and the SGB V (Social Security Code) were modified by the patients' rights law which came into effect on February 26, 2013 (Chaps. 2 and 15).

In this context, the Federal Joint Committee had to determine (until February 26, 2014) essential measures in its guidelines for internal quality management (as mentioned in § 137 section 1d Social Code V) to improve patients' safety, in particular minimum standards for RM systems

and fault reporting systems (Krystek and Fiege 2013).

In the future, hospitals shall also report on the implementation of RM and fault reporting systems in their quality report (according to section 3 no. 4 Patients' Rights Law 2013). The regulations for quality reports in hospitals have to be adapted accordingly by the Federal Joint Committee (FJC). This FJC development clearly shows that the legislator increasingly promotes efficient RM systems and transparency of fault culture. The consequences for developing the framework with minimum standards and remunerative models for participating in fault reporting systems between different institutions have to be approached.

20.3   Status of the Introduction to RM

In 2010, the Institute for Patient Safety – mandated by the Alliance for Patient Safety with the support of the AOK federal association – conducted a survey on German hospitals about the status concerning the introduction of clinical RM (Lauterbach et al. 2012):

> 484 hospitals (establishments) from 1,815 addressed clinics took part in the survey, representing a response rate of only 26.7 %. This number suggests that RM is still not widely implemented.

According to these survey results, one has to raise the following questions:

- *Are the goals and strategies for a clinical RM sufficiently defined?*
- *Which methods for gathering information about risks were used?*
- *How did risk analysis and resulting measures for risk minimization take place?*
- *Which methods for risk controlling were applied?*
- *What actions in the clinical RM were conducted within the scope of a continuous improvement process and how did documentation take place?*

- *How does handling with improvement requirements and professional needs take place?*
- *Are RM systems implemented as a PDCA
  system?*

The final report of the study published in 2012
shows that clinical RM is an issue in German
hospitals. This may not hide the fact that there is
still a significant potential for improvement of
operational introduction and implementation in
RM systems: Only about half of the hospitals
which took part in the survey introduced a defined
basic RM system. This is more surprising as the
provisions of the Commercial Code required by
every company, including hospitals, ensue an
accurate management.

The following consideration can basically be
deduced regarding to an assessment of this
survey:

Around 50 % of the 483 hospitals (sample,
1,815) have introduced a basic structure for an
RM system which is corresponding to approx.
242 clinics (13.4 %) of the proportionate sample.
If one assumes that the nonparticipating hospitals
in this survey have not introduced an RM system,
there is a significant backlog in the consensus of
the patient's, as well as the employee's interest,
for the introduction of an RM system.

20.4 RM – Quality Management – Fault Management

The term RM is often mentioned in the same
breath with quality management and fault management. In many hospitals, RM is organization-
ally and functionally positioned within the
quality management and is therefore understood
as part of quality management (Klein 2011).

The PDCA cycle which describes the stages
in the process of continuous improvement and
is the basis of all quality systems includes a
consistent fault management. The three terms
are therefore closely connected; however, a distinction still makes sense. While quality management is intended to improve quality and
efficiency of processes, the primary objective of

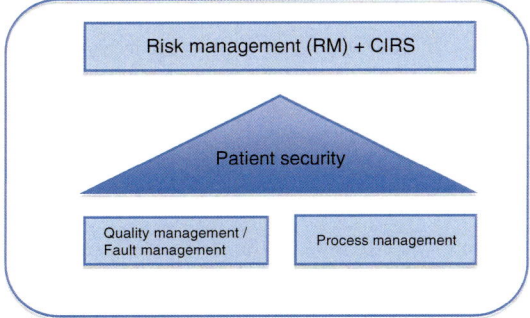

Fig. 20.2 Key elements for a successful patient
security (Source: own figure)

RM is to deal effectively with potential mistakes
before they occur – therefore, it has a prospective function (Klein 2011). It is obvious that
this increases the overall quality of an operating
hospital.

As shown in Fig. 20.2, RM in hospitals should
have an independent status.

The practice shows that patient safety can
only be achieved if RM is supported by quality
management and if hospitals adapt their processes to the respective requirements in a patient-
oriented way as well as adjusted to their risks.

To ensure improvements, a stabilization process must join the PDCA cycle (SDCA cycle:
standardize, do, check, act). Therefore, the standards for improving patient safety must also be
established (Kostka 2008).

20.5 RM and Planned Treatment Procedures

RM is not an isolated approach, and it should
involve all employees and processes of a hospital (Gaussmann 2007). It represents a comprehensive coverage, i.e., all areas of the hospital,
outpatient discharges, inpatient admissions, nursing ward, operation wards, specialist departments, administration, etc. The documentation
and establishment of treatment pathways shall
lead to the improvement of safety for patients
and staff and to risk reduction through optimization of processes and improved structures. This
inevitably leads to the consumption of hospital

resources, which in turn requires more money to be provided. In view of the tight budgets and accounting imbalances in many hospitals, that may be an obstacle for the introduction of RM.

One of the key areas of a hospital is the surgery ward. Especially here, an optimal use of resources and increase of efficiency is important. Within the framework of the operational management, individual steps inside the operating room will be analyzed, and inefficiencies will be detected in order to achieve an optimum resource allocation (*see* Chap. 10). In addition to the increase of efficiency, a possible improvement of quality should be implemented in the treatment process. The patient-centered treatment pathways must be highlighted with the perspective of possible emerging risks. In doing so, experiences from past claims of liability insurers can be included in the review, in order to use the resulting measures, if a remodeling of the patient-centered treatment pathways will be necessary.

As a first step of implementing an RM within the organization for operations, the benchmark hospital has to organize its flow structures on the basis of a potential hospital risk analysis:

(a) Operating areas, including recovery room
(b) Central admission
(c) Intensive care unit
(d) Other functional areas
(e) Areas for inpatient care
(f) Discharge management

Security checklists for surgery are already used in the operating rooms (OR) and were developed systematically to avoid faults (DGCH et al. 2009). In this project for implementing RM, error-prone problem areas are identified along with the perioperative process (Fig. 20.3).

The following sources of risks were taken into consideration:

P1:   Incomplete findings in the assessment requirements and insufficient documentation of patient records
P2:   Incorrect records on patients, missing or incomplete list of all ingested drugs, and nonobservance of interactive spectra in the case of premedications

P3:   Incorrect indications and insufficient information (lack of written documentation of information, missing signatures on the information sheet, information not in time)
P4:   Insufficient information on anesthesia
P5:   Incorrect planning of resources for the operational teams and incomplete planning for surgical operations (missing data)
P6:   Faulty care and transfer of patients (mistaken identity)
P7:   Sign in – allergies not recognized, respiration difficulty, and danger of blood loss
P8:   Time out – predictable critical incidents, antibiotic prophylaxis, and visible diagnostic imaging
P9:   Sign out – final check by nursing staff, surgeon, and anesthesia
P10/P11: Logistical problems (insufficient number of beds) on ward/intensive care unit
P12: Complete documents for patient transfer and organization of transport

Following clinic-related effects could be objectified by the implementation of this risk-adjusted PDCA cycle:

(a) Patient turnover in the operation arena was improved.
(b) The average waiting time of anesthetized patients could be lowered which reduces the risk of anesthesia for the patients.
(c) The number of patients for whom the surgery had to be canceled due to missing documents was reduced in the interest of the patients.
(d) Number of surgeries planned for a single shift which extended into the on-call service was lowered.
(e) Employee satisfaction increased through indications of an improvement in the failure rate of the operating room staff.
(f) Postoperative complication rates in patient care have been fortunately lowered.

A further development changing process will deal with the admission management: The area of hospital reference and discharge is especially fault prone due to interface issues. In this area, the hospital internal operating procedures for the benchmark hospital are currently being

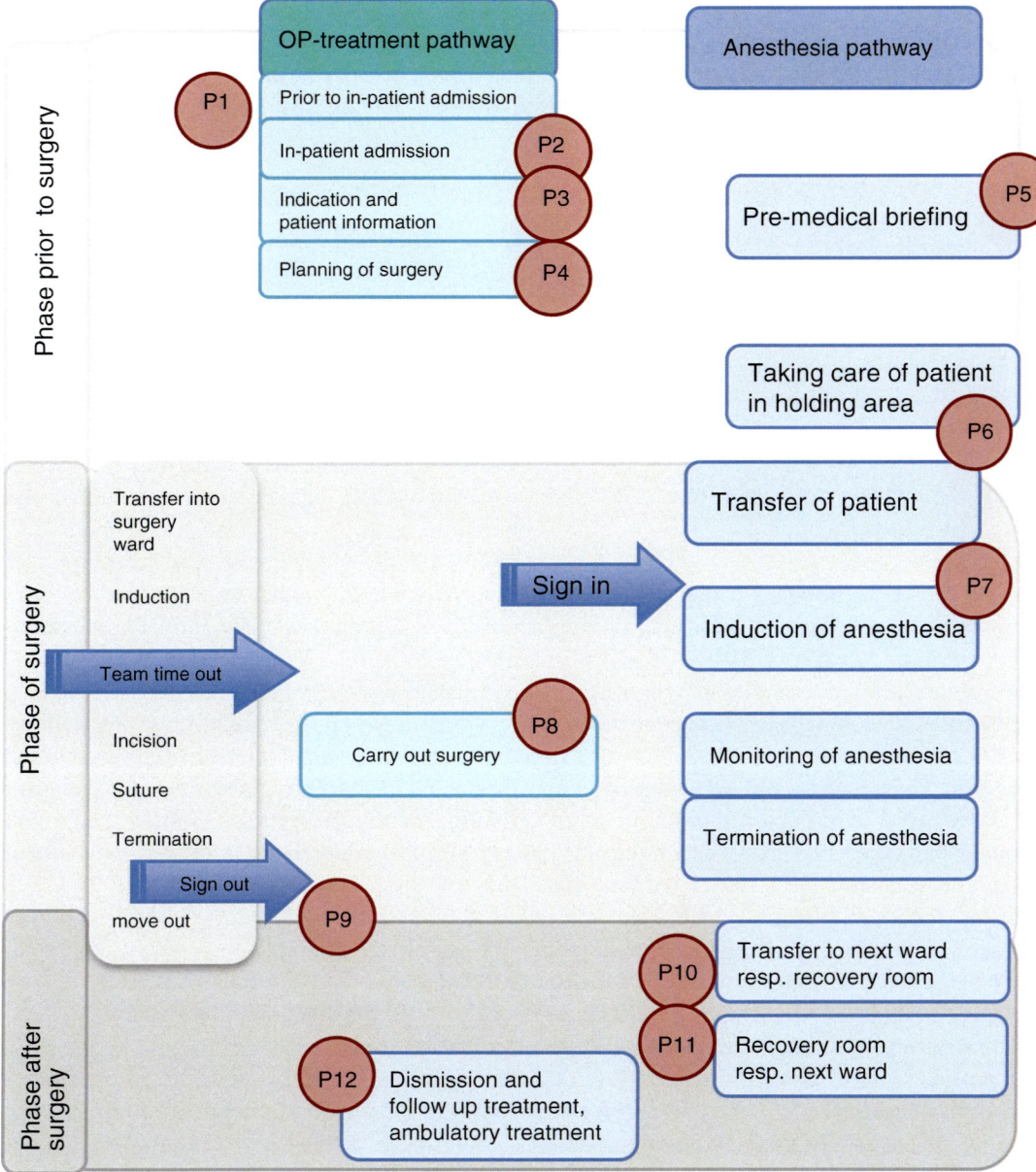

Fig. 20.3 Treatment pathways for operations (Source: own figure)

revised, taking into account the "checklists for medical interface management between the sectors of the health-care system (outpatient/inpatient treatment sectors)" (ÄZQ 2012). This is one of the major challenges for a best patient-orientated "full-diagnosed-based therapy." Consequently, near-missed therapy faults can be minimized.

20.6 Fault Management and CIRS

Chapter 9 *explains the method of the CIRS in detail*.

CIRS is to be understood as reporting and learning systems (Gunkel et al. 2013). Incident reporting systems can be integrated as a software solution by some providers into existing hospital information systems, but it is also possible to choose a web-based version, but also a paper-based system is possible (Gunkel et al. 2013).

CIRS – properly applied – will help the staff of the hospital to identify, analyze, and evaluate possible risks and near misses at an early stage.

In addition to the report feature, it is, however, crucial that CIRS is understood as a learning system, which means the findings obtained from the CIRS must result in the fault protection measures and lead to an adaptation of the work processes – only in this way a sustainable improvement for patient safety can be achieved.

20.6.1 How Does an Avoidable Incident Occur?

The safety barriers installed within a company are porous so that some of these safety barriers can be overcome through faults – *Reason* (1997) compares this fact with the holes in Swiss cheese. Usually successive safety barriers prevent that the error has consequences.

As the "Swiss cheese model" (*already presented in* Chap. 4 *of this book*) shows, a concatenation of unforeseen incidents and influencing factors can penetrate the security barriers and lead to an undesirable result.

All reports must be made primarily on a voluntary basis; thus, it is the responsibility of the employees whether they have reported on an incident or not. Nevertheless, all employees have to be informed and at least convinced through training courses about the benefit of a CIRS message. Therefore, the threshold for fault reporting is low if it is guaranteed that such missed incident reports are anonym. It must be fundamentally ensured in a hospital, despite the limited number of hospital employees who may be taken into consideration for the near miss, that employees shall be protected in their privacy.

Only when this personal anonymity of an individual employee in a hospital can be preserved, a CIRS will successfully lead to a higher transparency in patient and employee safety! This requires a new culture, whereby a high level of trust exists between the employees. By these means, the anonymity will be indispensable.

For this purpose, a neutral registration office in the hospital must be established which works on, analyzes, and evaluates the CIRS reports; sometimes this happens centrally in corporations.

It is important that the lessons learned from the CIRS messages are made transparent to the employees, i.e., by changes in the process, where corporations and also partner clinics can be viewed. Normally, this will have a positive and motivating effect to participate in CIRS. Only through a proactive commitment on behalf of the staff can CIRS lead, in the long-term, to an improvement of patient and employee safety.

It is important that the reporting process systematically operates in a user-friendly way. When working with a computer-based solution, the masks have to be user-friendly and intuitive in order to leave brief messages, if necessary, and especially working under time pressure. In addition, it is essential that the form for messages must be consistent to make a comparative examination and assessment possible.

Under legal consideration, no cases shall be reported that resulted in patient injury, which then could lead, where appropriate, into a lawsuit (Höfinger et al. 2008; Paula 2007). In such cases, the supervisor has to be informed who will in turn inform the *hospital management.*

20.6.2 How Could a Fault Culture in Hospital Be Enhanced?

One approach to the development of a fault culture in hospital is shown in Fig. 20.4 (see below).

The advancement of a confidence building culture in a clinic begins at the top with the management. Here, the managerial staff of each department must first develop confidence building measures within the framework of a workshop. That will have a signal effect on the employees.

At departmental levels, team rulings have to be defined that support a respectful way in dealing with each other and do not allow for denunciation. This culture must be lived up to, and readjustments, if necessary, should be made by an accompanying evaluation.

Finally, a written employee survey should be carried out according to a defined period of

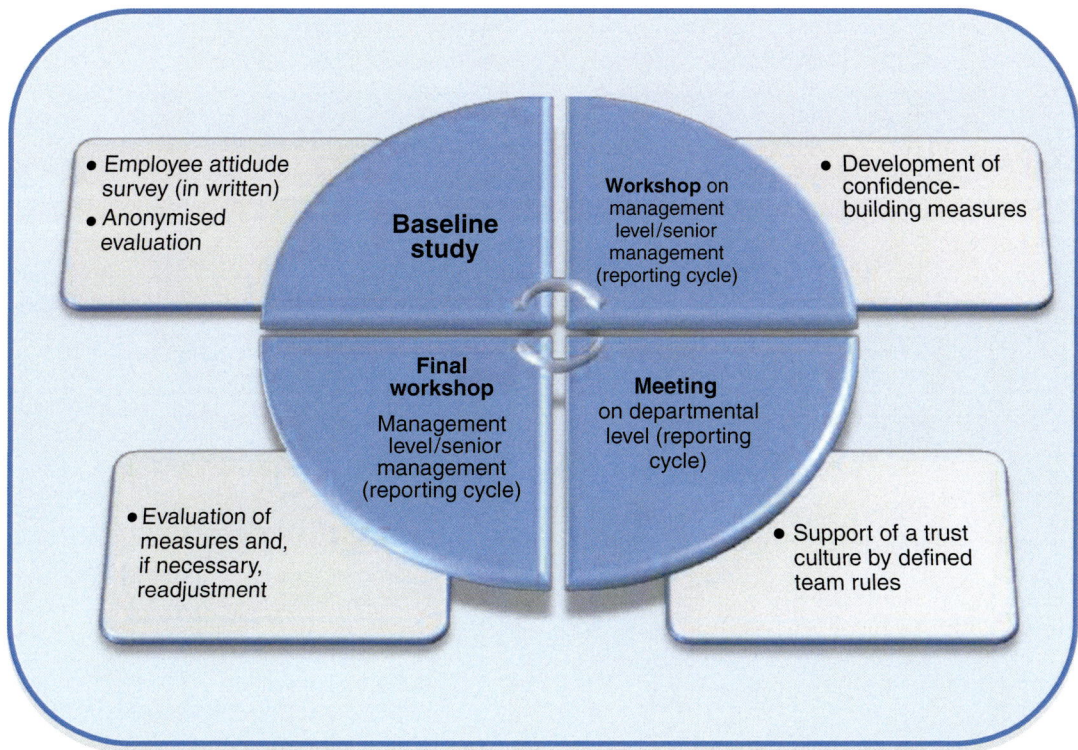

Fig. 20.4 Practical procedures for further development of a fault culture (Source: own figure adapted to R. Heuzeroth 2012, Asklepios Klinken)

time and then evaluated anonymously in order to assess whether progress can be recorded or not. It takes a long time to establish a safe fault culture in the minds of the employees – in terms of improving patient safety – however, it is definitely worthwhile to follow through with it.

20.6.3 The Psychological Aspects to Establish a CIRS Must Therefore Be Observed

The introduction of CIRS in hospitals takes place according to the procedure of a classical project management (see Fig. 20.5), *see also* Chap. 19. To ensure a structured approach, a project plan must be created on behalf of the management cycle of the hospital in which the individual sub-objectives are defined with the corresponding milestones. In regard to the RM and CIRS process, there are, among others, recommendations for a structured approach published

by the German Alliance for Patient Safety (Aktionsbündnis Patientensicherheit 2007).

This structured approach saves resources and money which are usually scarce.

The benchmark hospital has achieved its first important results through the planning, implementation and pilot phase in the surgical field which now requires readjustments within the scope of further process optimization. Concerning other areas of the hospital there are still a number of large steps required before such a RM system is available nationwide in all hospitals.

20.7   Summary

Above all, a fault reporting system will only be successful if it is regarded as an integral part of an efficient RM and CIRS that is accompanied with a patient-centered process management.

However, the following considerations should be respected which are associated with

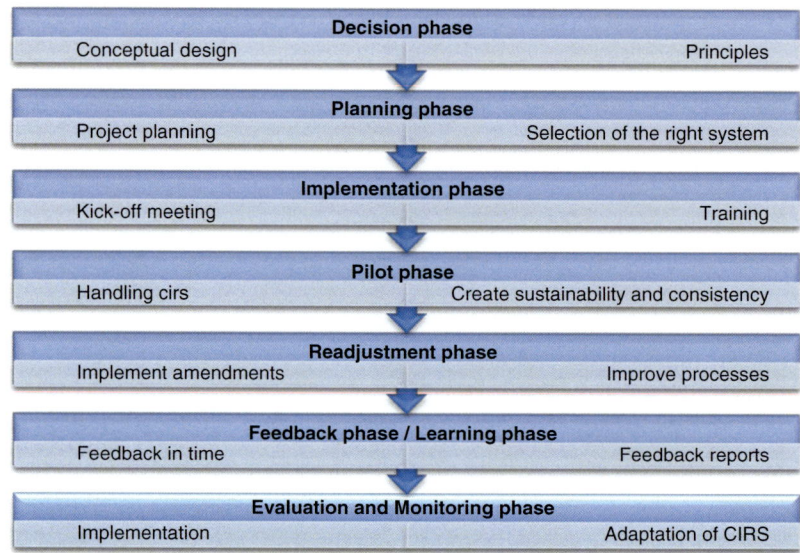

Fig. 20.5 Recommendations on how to proceed in introducing CIRS in hospital (Source: own figure according to the German Alliance for Patient Safety)

an RM system that is actively realized by the total hospital staff:

(a) An existing high level of medical performance will be improved by further fault prevention.
(b) Patient safety will be increased.
(c) Protection of the hospital staff will be increased avoiding possible missed or realized treatment failures, especially regarding the intensified, higher working load in patient care.
(d) Patient-centered treatment processes require a sufficient acknowledgement for employees to fulfill their profession ethics.
(e) Finally, a working RM and CIRS optimize the resource management.

Bibliography

Aktionsbündnis Patientensicherheit (2007) Empfehlungen zur Einführung von Critical Incident Reporting Systemen (CIRS)
ÄZQ (2012) Checklisten für das ärztliche Schnittstellenmanagement zwischen den Versorgungssektoren, 1.Auflage

DGCH, Sicherheits-Checkliste Chirurgie, Globale Initiative für Patientensicherheit, deutsche Adaptation von Haynes AB, Weiser TG, Berry WR et al (2009) A surgical safety checklist to reduce morbidity and mortality in a global population. NEJM 360:491–498
Krystek and Fiege (2013) Risikomanagement, Gabler Wirtschaftslexikon. http://wirtschaftslexikon.gabler.de/Archiv/7669/risikomanagement-v9.html
Gaussmann P (2007) Risikomanagement und geplante Behandlungspfade, Schriftenreihe Gesundheitswirtschaft Band 2 Risikomanagement, 2.Auflage, S.207–201
Gesetz zur Verbesserung der Rechte von Patientinnen und Patienten, Artikel 2 Abs.8, Bundesgesetzblatt 2013 Teil1 Nur.9
Gunkel C et al (2013) CIRS-Gemeinsames Lernen durch Berichts- und Lernsysteme, ÄZQ Schriftenreihe 42
Heuzeroth R (2012) CIRS, 2.Nationales CIRS-Forum Berlin
Hoffmann B (2010) Patientensicherheit und Fehlermanagement: Ursachen unerwünschter Ereignisse und Maßnahmen zu ihrer Vermeidung. Dtsch. Ärzteblatt 3:23
Höfinger G, Horstmann R, Wahlrzek H (2008) Das Lernen aus Zwischenfällen lernen: Incident Reporting im Krankenhaus, Gabler Verlag, Buchkapitel, S.207–224
Klein A (2011) Risikomanagement und Risiko-Controlling. Haufeverlag, S. 225–230
Kostka C (2008) Der kontinuierliche Verbesserungsprozess: Methoden des KVP, 4.Auflage. Hanser Verlag, S.38
Lauterbach K et al (2012) Abschlussbericht: Befragung zum Einführungsstand von klinischem

Risikomanagement in deutschen Krankenhäusern.. Institut für Patientensicherheit, Bonn

Paula H (2007) Patientensicherheit und Risikomanagement im Pflege- und Krankenhausalltag, Springer Verlag, S.91–92

Reason J (1997) Managing the risks of organizational accidents. Ashgate Publishing, Hampshire

Riedel R, Schmidt S, Bauer H (2013) Patientenrechtegesetz und die Folgen für das Risikomanagement. Dt Ärzteblatt 110(1–2):A-14

Further Reading

Collins M (2009) On the prospects for a blame-free medical culture. Soc Sci Med 69(9):1287–1290

Cooper J (1996) Is voluntary reporting of critical events effective for quality assurance? Anesthesiology 85(5): 961–964

Dunn D (2003) Incident reports Correcting – processes and reducing errors. AORN J 78(2). doi:http://dx.doi.org/10.1016/S0001-2092(06)60772-2

Hogan H et al (2008) What can we learn about patient safety from information sources within an acute hospital: a step on the ladder of integrated risk management? Qual Saf Health Care 17:209–215. doi:10.1136/qshc.2006.020008

Kohn LT, Corrigan J, Donaldson MS (2000) Institute of medicine (US), committee on quality of health care in America. To err is human: building a safer health care system. National Academy of Sciences, Washington, DC

Leape L (2002) Reporting of adverse events. N Engl J Med 347(20):1633–1638

Mahajan R (2010) Critical incident reporting and learning. Br J Anaesth 105(1):69–75. doi:10.1093/bja/aeq133

Riedel R, Schmidt S (2013) Patientenrechtegesetz 2013: Was Ärzte und Management beachten müssen. Krankenhaus und Management

Riedel R, Schulenburg D (2011) Wichtige Gesetze im Gesundheitswesen. NWB

Vincent C, Taylor-Adams S, Stanhope N (1998) Framework for analysing risk and safety in clinical medicine. BMJ 316(7138):1154–1157

Vincent C, Taylor-Adams S, Chapman EJ, Hewett D (2000) How to investigate and analyse clinical incidents: Clinical Risk Unit and Association of Litigation and Risk Management protocol. BMJ 320. doi:http://dx.doi.org/10.1136/bmj.320.7237.777

World Alliance for Patient Safety (2005) WHO draft guidelines for adverse event reporting and learning systems: from information to action. World Health Organization, Geneva, Available from: http://www.who.int/patient-safety/events/05/Reporting_Guidelines.pdf

Sonja Sieger

Abstract

Since ancient times, people are working on the idea of quality. The goal is to create standards of quality. Since then, numerous systems and tools have been developed with many different operating divisions and units. Rising quality requirements result in lower liability risks. In this context, quality has a great financial relevance. Demands for quality assurance in medicine and healthcare have been enforced in the past. For the purposes of the patient and in the context of globalization, it is increasingly necessary to ensure comparable quality in healthcare all over the world. Already in 2005 with the CEN/TS 15224, a guide was developed that sets out requirements for quality management systems in medicine and healthcare. For medical and healthcare services, the first national and European-wide recognized certifiable standard was adopted in October 2012 with the DIN EN 15224. The framework has the potential to found international recognition.

21.1 A History of Quality

Even in ancient times, people were concerned with quality considerations and the aim of creating quality standards. When it comes to architecture and quality assurance in construction, the Code of Hammurabi saw the development and publication of framework specifications intended to ensure quality and prevent hazards as many as 3700 years ago. Many years later, as quality concepts for space travel and electrotechnology were developed, probabilities and statistical possibilities were increasingly referred to.

In 1961 the "zero-defect program" emerged from the development and production of new rocket systems for the US Army, but it was not until around 20 years later that Western industry became aware that quality and quality management need to be taken into account as a decisive factor for positioning in competition. Demands for suppliers to adhere to and certify quality criteria were defined, initially emanating from NATO and then from NASA. See also Chap. 14 for the development history of the concept of quality.

S. Sieger
TÜV PROFiCERT-Lead Auditorin,
TÜV Technische Überwachung Hessen GmbH,
Managementsysteme, Rüdesheimer str. 119,
Darmstadt 64285, Germany
e-mail: sonja.sieger@tuevhessen.de

© Springer-Verlag Berlin Heidelberg 2016
W. Merkle (ed.), *Risk Management in Medicine*, DOI 10.1007/978-3-662-47407-5_21

With its "Allied Quality Assurance Publications," NATO defined criteria for the first time, in line with which suppliers had to certify their ability to assure quality. This certification gave the suppliers a significant competitive and market advantage. The development resulted in many industrial sectors picking up on the concept of quality.

William Edwards Deming (1900–1993), considered as a pioneer of quality management, developed the Deming or PDCA (plan, do, check, act) cycle and expanded the concept of quality beyond the production industry to ultimately include service fields too. Deming focused his work on continuous improvement processes and the associated management of risks. The PDCA cycle is the most important foundation of the continuous improvement process, making it a key basis for relevant standards in quality management (see also Chaps. 1 and 6).

Since then, many systems and tools (see Chap. 6 and the specialist chapters on CIRS, OTAS, TTO, etc.) have been developed and incorporated into a wide range of corporate divisions and specialist fields.

21.2   Quality in Medicine and Healthcare

Healthcare facilities have to manage on a very limited budget and are under increasing economic pressure. Quality management is becoming more and more important in order to prevent the quality of treatment from suffering under purely economic specifications and against the background of reducing liability and risk as well as protecting against organizational fault. The reduced liability risks resulting from this mean that fewer reserves are needed and are therefore relevant from a financial point of view (cf. Chap. 20).

Quality saves costs: Statistics have shown that poor quality and errors in healthcare in particular lead to the need for follow-up treatment and thus cause unnecessary additional costs. A rethink is required. Dr. Robert Califf, cardiac specialist at the Duke University Medical Center,

commented in *The New York Times* on how his colleagues deal with errors that are made public: "It is just like the stages of grief described by death researcher Kübler-Ross in connection with impending death: The person who is about to die is first in shock, then denial, and finally he accepts the idea."

Some calls for quality assurance in medicine and healthcare have already gained both national and international acceptance in the form of regulatory requirements. In addition, significant efforts are being made to represent the quality of results and care using statistics in "quality registers," thus creating transparency, such as in the work of the Hospital Quality Alliance (HQA) in the USA. Participating hospitals receive financial support from health insurance providers in setting up a QM system. HQA has already led to improvements in the quality of patient care in the USA. In the UK, the statistics are presented via the NHS Choices portal, where staff also has the chance to judge their own facility. Denmark gives public warnings about poor doctors.

In Germany, the AQUA-Institute publishes quality reports on behalf of the Federal Joint Committee (G-BA), which is demanding mandatory risk management and error notification systems in 2014 in order to improve patient safety in relation to independent doctors, dentists, and hospitals.

When combined with gathering, analyzing, and evaluating quality-relevant data and indicators, quality management is the prospective basis for appropriate quality of results. Quality management is oriented toward the whole organization and its processes and aims to safeguard quality systematically. Quality assurance, quality management, as well as risk and error management are mutually dependent on one another and can reasonably not be considered isolated from each other. The focus of quality management in the healthcare sector is on systematically checking and controlling processes and minimizing, or ideally eliminating, avoidable clinical risks, for the benefit of the patient and patient safety as well as benefit and safety of the staff and the hospital as a company.

Internal quality management incorporates normative, statutorily prescribed, and internal company regulations and measures equally.

A wide range of regulations with a more or less quality-relevant background has developed both nationally and internationally in recent times. However, often shaped by interest groups, funders, and lobbyists, the regulations have so far often caused confusion and resentment. The development is as yet no closer to achieving the goal of ensuring international uniform minimum standards in healthcare.

This background makes creating regulations and having adherence to the relevant requirements monitored by independent bodies particularly important.

21.3   Monitoring by External Bodies

Conformity assessment and certification bodies are responsible for assessing and monitoring the conformity of companies – their services, products, systems, and processes – with the relevant requirements from standards, directives, and laws. A conformity assessment by an independent body transparently shows third parties whether and to what extent an organization conforms to the relevant requirements and regulations and implements them internally.

Quality and certainty in reliability and achieved results of the assessments predominantly depend on the body conducting the assessment using appropriate specialist expertise and a qualified process. As part of accreditation (accredit < lat. > believe), certification bodies have to demonstrate their competence and a qualified process in line with the requirements of DIN EN ISO/IEC 17011 and DIN EN ISO/IEC 17021 to the accreditation body responsible in the respective country.

"Accredited certification bodies" recognized by the accreditation body responsible in the respective country (such as TÜV Hessen, DQS, etc.) are constantly monitored.

One focus is on high standards for the impartiality and objectivity of the certification body,

including the staff involved. When conducting certification audits in the accredited segment, accredited certification bodies only use staff who meets the specifications defined in DIN EN ISO 19011.

Internationally, agreements on conformity assessment programs in the management system, product, service, and person sectors are steered by the International Accreditation Forum (IAF).

Some of the medicine and healthcare standards developed by lobbyists are thought to contain a conflict of interest in terms of quality and patient safety and are subject to critical scrutiny with respect to their objectivity and independence.

21.4   WHO Demands International Coordination

The European Committee for Standardization has already been working on a single standard for quality management in the healthcare sector, corresponding to the latest expertise, for over a decade.

Already 30 years ago, the World Health Organization (WHO) was calling loudly for attempts to be made at an internationally coordinated quality management system for medicine and healthcare. Quite apart from the fundamental benefits of a system like this, the interests of the patient and the background of globalization are making it ever more essential that comparable quality in healthcare is going to be ensured.

In addition, interdisciplinary cooperation in the consistent adherence to minimum requirements is becoming more and more important, as a range of specialist disciplines and organizations are increasingly involved in the patient's recovery process.

Statutory requirements and funders have had some success in demanding quality management within healthcare facilities over the past few years. However, national or even international coordination of the systems has failed so far.

There is no recognized set of regulations that defines a minimum standard of this kind.

21.5   DIN EN ISO 9001

The technical committee ISO/TC 176 was founded in 1980 and began passing the ISO 9000 series of standards in 1987. The first version of DIN EN ISO 9001 came into effect in 2008 and remains the basis for existing certifications to this day. It will be revised and reissued in 2015.

21.6   CEN/TS 15224:2005

As early as 2005, the CEN/TS 15224 saw the development of guidelines governing the requirements for quality management systems in medicine and healthcare.

It was worked on by the European Committee for Standardization (CEN), with the cooperation of German quality experts, the German Institute for Standardization (DIN) and the Standards Committee Medical (NAMed), and developed into a standard suitable for certification purposes.

As well as its role in certification, the standard is also suitable as a guideline for systematically establishing, maintaining, and further developing a quality management system. Currently the first of its kind to be recognized both nationally and across Europe, the standard can be used for certification and was passed in October 2012 as DIN EN 15224.

This is a revolutionary and long overdue development.

21.7   DIN EN 15224:2012

The development of sets of regulations like this originates in the intention to manage entire companies, processes, and risks and to create a fundament for comparable quality. Considering the company as a whole and thinking outside the box are among others the most important bases for steering an organization and managing avoidable risks.

Looking at the set of regulations, the relationship to the aforementioned DIN EN ISO 9001 – the "mother of all standards" – is impossible to miss. Risk management is demanded in every chapter of 15224 and also includes documentation, responsibility for performance, human resources, work environment, infrastructure, scientific divisions (development), purchasing process, supplier requirements, and clinical processes themselves.

The principle and structure of EN 15224 are based on the proven ISO 9001. Healthcare organizations considered the production-related origin as "difficult to accept" and often as unfit for their purpose. In contrast, EN 15224 speaks about patients and clinical processes and specifies the requirements for service providers in healthcare. Just like its "mother," the standard can be applied to subdivisions, apart from certification of the entire organization.

The standard incorporates the international classification (ICF), as well as taking specific regulatory requirements into account. It is oriented toward primary care, prehospital care, hospital nursing, tertiary care, nursing homes, hospices, preventative healthcare, psychiatric care, dental health services, physiotherapy, occupational health services, rehabilitation, and pharmacies.

Apart from the normative requirements for the organization, 11 clearly defined quality characteristics provide the benchmark for the requirements in Chapters 4 to 8. Preconditions and interactions specific to healthcare are also incorporated into the set of regulations. Already familiar and proven from ISO 9001, the process-oriented approach relates to all clinical processes, research, training, and its risk management.

Just like its "mother," the standard is structured in eight main chapters.

Its content is oriented toward clinical processes and the language is adapted accordingly. The summary of the content given below is intended as an overview and does not claim to be exhaustive.

In addition to providing general information and normative references, Chapters 0 to 3 of EN 15224 define the scope and explain special terms.

The quality characteristics for healthcare services are defined as follows:
- Appropriate, correct care
- Availability
- Continuity of care
- Effectiveness
- Efficiency
- Egality
- Evidence- and knowledge-based care
- Care oriented toward the patient, including physical, psychological, and social integrity
- Inclusion of the patient
- Patient safety
- Timeliness and accessibility

The normative requirements for the organization are governed in Chapters 4 to 8.

21.8 Quality Management Systems

Chapter 4 defines the requirements for the quality management system.

The chapter contains general requirements for the organization and basic documentation requirements. The standard demands that the organization's quality policy and objectives are documented. The scope, documented processes including clinical processes and risks, and a description of how individual processes interact are to be documented within the quality management manual.

Clinical and other processes must be recognized and defined in line with the quality requirements stated above. As part of this, indicators, criteria, and methods for assessment shall be defined, and appropriate measures shall be taken. The process for dealing with clinical risks must be depicted. These regulations, including how to deal with potential risks, also relate to outsourced processes and services and must therefore also be applied to external staff or those under contract.

The chapter demands that documents, such as clinical guidelines, logs, operating instructions, checklists, medical device manuals, and documents relating to clinical risks and management, are steered systematically. Staff entrusted with the relevant competencies must be enabled to assess, update, and steer documentation of this kind.

21.9 Management Responsibility

Chapter 5 governs the responsibility of management. As part of the quality management system, top management is obliged to conduct constant development, implementation, and improvement. The effectiveness of the entire system with regard to regulatory and official requirements, the quality characteristics, and patient expectations is to be ensured at management level. The standard demands commitments on quality policy and objectives and incorporates the entire company, individual divisions and processes, and risk management.

Going beyond the basic of customer orientation, Chapter 5 demands requirements on responsibility, authority, internal communication, and its documentation.

The management must review the management system at planned intervals. This must include process performance, such as morbidity or mortality, the results of internal audits, customer feedback, and the status of preventive actions, corrective actions, as well as risk management. In addition, the assessment must include regulatory requirements and the efficiency of outsourced processes. The results of the management review shall lead to decisions and measures being taken to improve the system and processes, including in the form of customer requirements and new approaches to clinical processes.

A management representative must be nominated, entrusted with coordinating the quality work, and equipped with the appropriate resources and authority and knowledge.

21.10 Management of Resources

Chapter 6 defines the provision and management of resources, including regulations on HR resources, the infrastructure and, the working environment. The organization must also provide auxiliary services, including appropriate information and communication systems, in this context.

Fundamental requirements for the qualification and competence of the staff, as well as awareness of the quality characteristics and risks enshrined in the standard and the associated necessity of training, are demanded. Apart from the availability, sustainability, and reliability of the relevant resources, any clinical risks that occur must be analyzed, and this analysis must result in concepts being defined. The organization must ensure that the staff implement services in an evidence- and knowledge-based way for all areas of activity and clinical processes and incorporate management of clinical risks into this.

Clinical risks must also be analyzed and assessed once again as part of the infrastructure requirements. Put simply, an available, sustainable, and reliable infrastructure must be guaranteed, taking medical products, other equipment, and supporting services into account.

21.11 Providing the Service in Healthcare

Chapter 7 is dedicated to providing the service.

Relevant processes have to be identified and systematically governed.

This requirement concerns customer-related processes, development, procurement, service provision, and steering monitoring and measurement means.

As part of providing services, the sector-specific quality criteria set out in the standard and the regulatory requirements must be adhered to. The patient must be involved in determining and assessing requirements for clinical processes. Clinical and knowledge-based standards and findings, regulatory requirements, and requirements from financing organizations must be incorporated into the planning, implementation, and assessment.

The standard demands requirements on communication with the patient and suggests details on processes, costs, benefits, possible complications, side effects, alternative treatments, and the length of treatment. Regulations regarding how patients' property is handled must be made and be applied in the organization.

Development processes such as the application of new procedures within clinical processes or clinical trials must be planned and assessed under consideration of the development input. The same as design and development processes, the processes for service provision and purchasing have to be verified and validated in adherence to the documentation requirements.

As part of implementing the services, the standard demands a process for the labeling and traceability of the patient, clinical processes, devices and materials, as well as the staff involved. The way medical devices, pharmaceuticals, and similar things are handled must also be governed in this context.

21.12 Measurement, Analysis, and Improvement

Chapter 8 defines measurement, analysis, and improvement within the organization. This takes into account customers (patients, relatives, interested parties) and suppliers on the one hand and internal audits and the monitoring and measurement of clinical processes and risks on the other. As part of customer satisfaction, the organization shall define methods that can be used to find out the extent to which customer requirements are met.

At this point, the standard demands that measures for improving patient safety are labeled and implemented systematically.

Concepts and documentation regarding the process for dealing with a missing service and corrective as well as preventative actions are also required.

In addition, the chapter demands the analysis, recording, and transparency of clinical processes, clinical risks, near misses, events, and unwanted incidents. Documented concepts for implementing corrective and preventative actions must be made available and must incorporate clinical risks and continuous improvement.

The entire regulation can be obtained from Beuth Verlag: www.beuth.de.

21.13   Implementation of DIN EN 15224

The very best aspect of EN 15224 is clearly Attachment B, in which the standard provides sector-specific information on the practical implementation of the standard's demands in simple language.

21.14   Summary and Forecast

Service providers in healthcare already conduct their activities against a backdrop of regulatory requirements, as well as having to meet the standards of their funders. In this sense, the normative demands appear to offer little in terms of new content. Despite this, enormous differences in quality can be seen between the individual providers of healthcare services, both on a national and international level. Pay for performance (P4P) is one possible strategy for making quality more interesting from an economic point of view. Clear national regulations on the proportional assumption of costs for quality management, risk management, and quality assurance also appear sensible and necessary.

As P4P may overtax small rural hospitals which however are mandatory for medical service reachable for patients also in thinly populated areas, external support in risk management implementation might be necessary.

The quality of the healthcare service throughout the entire treatment process is no longer determined by a single "treater" today. Given this agreement, safeguarding the quality of results depends on all service providers involved in the entire process adhering to the relevant requirements. This requires defining and adhering to uniform minimum requirements for all service providers involved in the treatment process.

Over 30 years after the WHO's demand, a foundation for a harmonized quality management system in medicine and healthcare has been created nationally and (currently) across Europe.

EN 15224 has the potential to achieve broad recognition on an international level.

The standard defines fundamental minimum requirements for service providers in the healthcare sector in a set of requirements that can be used for certification. Risk management and error notification systems for improving patient safety relate to all normative requirements and are oriented toward the 11 defined quality characteristics.

The set of requirements allows institutions and services to be compared on the basis of minimum standards and this to be verified by independent third parties, i.e., accredited certification bodies (e.g., TÜV, DQS, etc.).

Link: http://www.tuev-hessen.de

More information (TÜV PROFiCERT Lead Auditor): sonja.sieger@tuevhessen.de

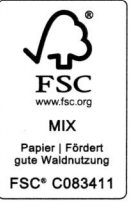
Zeitfracht Medien GmbH
Ferdinand-Jühlke-Straße 7
99095 Erfurt, Deutschland
produktsicherheit@kolibri360.de